Runner's World

YOGA
BOOK

Runner's World

YOGA BOOK

**by Jean Couch
with
Nell Weaver**

Runner's World Books

Library of Congress Cataloging in Publication Data

Couch, Jean M.
Runner's world yoga book.

Bibliography: p. 219
1. Yoga, Hatha. I. Runner's World. II. Title.
RA781.7.C68   613.7   78-68619
ISBN 0-89037-206-3 (spiral)
ISBN 0-89037-236-5 (perfectbound)
ISBN 0-89037-247-0 (hardbound)

Illustrations by Cheryl Valdin

Second printing July 1980
Third printing March 1981
New Edition 1982

© 1979 by
Jean M. Couch

Runner's World Books
1400 Stierlin Rd.
Mountain View, CA 94043

Contents

To Janie

Acknowledgments

I wish to acknowledge

First, the Grace that gave me the opportunity to write this book. I have enjoyed the experience enormously!

Second, the ultimate source of this information, Mr. B. K. S. Iyengar of Poona, India. I have unlimited respect for his genius and overflowing gratitude for his willingness to share it.

Third, Nell Weaver of Little Rock, Arkansas for her bountiful contributions, editorial and otherwise. Behind this author is an excellent contributor! Nell wishes to thank her teacher, Janet Downs.

Fourth, my teachers: Ramanand Patel, and the teachers at the Institute for Yoga Teacher Education in San Francisco; Felicity Hall, Mary Dunn, Larry Hatlett, Melinda Perlee, Bonita Bradley, Toni Montez, Judith Lasater, Bridgett Gleason.

Fifth, all my students. Each person brings his or her own mystery. Every person is an education.

Sixth, Dr. Gary Harper of Little Rock, Arkansas, for reading the physiology section. Emily Stewart, Los Altos, Calif., for reviewing the "Yoga on Your Own" section.

Seventh, my family. Whitney, 3, helped so much with her secretarial skills: sharpening pencils, walking on chapters, stapling everything in sight. Matthew, 6, for the jar of worms on my desk and his steadfast belief that indeed this would one day be over so we could go to the park again. Michael, husband, lover, friend, who pulled us all through with his even disposition, good humor and generosity. My Mom and Dad, Iva and Bill McWilliams, who spent all those years helping me prepare for such a satisfying project as this.

Preface

Here I am writing the first words last. It's wonderful to write a book because you can "let it rip" and say so many things you've always wanted to say. There's one final (initial?) thing I want to mention.

I wish I could include a dehydrated capsule; you add the water and out would come a miniature teacher. One to scream and yell at you, to cajole you, to direct you, to encourage you, to teach you yoga. One who would work you when you baby yourself, one to hold you back when you push too hard. One that has so much love and respect for you and for yoga that by his or her talents he or she helps you discover yourself.

But since I can't include this ultimate gimmick I plead with you to draw upon your imagination as you use this book. The pictures are static, the directions are precise, the intent is serious. But don't let the medium kill the humanity of it all. There will be times when you will want to laugh, cry, curse, quit. Do all of those things but then return. Return to the poses in this book and bit by bit you will indeed become flexible.

Flexibility is the ability to change. That's what we're after—the ability to see and adjust, see and adjust, see and adjust. Hatha yoga teaches flexibility through the concreteness of the body but the flexibility you gain will be much more than physical.

I wish I could shower you with my enthusiasm, to give you the spark of interest that will lead you to the discoveries possible through the practice of this marvelous scientific art form of the body, mind, spirit—YOGA!

PART ONE
THE BASICS

1

Eastern Yoga For The Western Athlete

The specialized ways of the Western world have so thoroughly dissected man that it has been common to accept false divisions of man into body, mind, and spirit. The emphasis on intellectual pursuits accompanied by rampant neglect of both body and spirit are manifestations of the assumption that happiness can be accomplished in the head alone. Signs of unrest with this situation are visible everywhere. Self-help and consciousness-raising groups are flourishing. Physical fitness has risen to new heights in status. These new waves of enthusiasm reflect the attempt to more thoroughly integrate the physical with the mental and spiritual. The East has dealt with this problem literally for centuries. For individuals to realize the wholeness of man the East devised yoga.

The word "yoga" means union or joining. There are numerous systems of yoga, each providing different ways to unify the various aspects of man. The yoga system this book deals with is hatha yoga. In the most simplistic terms, hatha yoga means yoga for health, the physical aspects of yoga. The word "hatha" implies balance: "ha" means sun and "tha" means moon. This system of yoga aims to balance—to join—different energy flows within the human body.

Hatha yoga is the system most familiar to the westerner. It works through the concreteness of the body. Hatha yoga uses physical poses to explore the inner structures of the body, the mind, and the self. It is a path, a guide, a step-by-step method that can lead you to greater self-knowledge. Each pose is a means to feel inwardly, to discover where you are strong, tight, weak, or dull. Hatha yoga provides the framework for the experiences of physical, mental, and spiritual wholeness.

Within the system of hatha yoga there are numerous schools, each following one person's teachings. This book's poses are based for the most part on the teaching of B. K. S. Iyengar. The Iyengar method emphasizes precise and careful body alignment, muscular balance, and maximum spinal extension. Therefore, this school of yoga is a science of postural work most useful to the western athlete.

Top athletes differ from other people in some predictable ways. Most superior athletes have balanced postural alignment and muscle tone. It stands to reason that if the average athlete can improve posture and maximize muscular balance, athletic performance will improve.

The Iyengar method of yoga is based on a central principle of balance. Physiologically, balance means several things. First, each individual muscle is capable of contracting, lengthening, and relaxing; second, corresponding muscle groups (for example, hamstrings and quadriceps) are equally strong and stretched; third, the joints, when surrounded by balanced muscle tissues, are free to move in their full range of motion; fourth, alignment of the body makes it possible to accommodate a full breath; and finally, energy flows equally to all parts of the body.

When the body is balanced, flesh feels like flesh; it is neither too hard (and susceptible to injury) nor too soft (and incapable of supporting the skeleton properly). When the body is balanced the skeletal-muscular system facilitates movement rather than hinders it, and the body is designed for nothing if not for movement. Balanced movement is self-perpetuating; the more freely you move the more you can move.

The Iyengar school of hatha yoga promotes this balance better than any other school of hatha yoga or any fitness information presently available. His system teaches how to move the spine to preserve and strengthen its God-given integrity. His is the only system that provides each student with specific instructions on how to nurture muscular balance and perfect posture. And the marvel of it all is that it works through the concreteness of the body. There is nothing magical or mystical. You don't have to believe a thing to experience yoga's benefits. What you must do is practice the poses. The means to physical, mental, and spiritual wholeness are your own body in the poses and your own willingness to observe closely how you feel. Athletes are already working with their bodies; what many need to do is learn a new way to look and to feel in order to bring about a more satisfying harmony that comes not only from physical equilibrium but from mental and spiritual balance as well.

2

Stretching Vs. Yoga

Stretching differs from yoga in process and purpose. Stretching is jerky and forced. Yoga poses are slow and controlled. Stretching aims for certain degrees of flexibility. Yoga aims for physical, mental, and spiritual balance.

Stretching has traditionally been taught using the *dynamic* or ballistic stretch. This means that a person bounces or jerks into a certain position. The completed stretch is seldom held for more than a few seconds. This method of stretching reflects the mental attempt to force the body to certain limits. People engaged in this type of activity are spurred on by what they see someone else do or by what someone else expects. They compare themselves to others and to goals others have set for them. Stretching in such cases is competitive.

Yoga, on the other hand, uses the *static* stretch. This means that a person uses a slow, steady motion to enter a pose and then holds at the limit of his or her stretch for ten seconds to ten minutes or longer. The slowness of yoga gives the practitioner greater control over the positioning, safety, and efficiency of each pose. This static stretch also makes it possible for a person to look within, to feel how she or he responds physically and emotionally to the poses. Yoga is introspective.

The intent of dynamic stretching is to achieve pre-determined degrees of flexibility. The attempt is made to force the body into a mold. The body is used as a tool to accomplish a specific goal.

The brain dictates to the body; there is little reciprocation between body and brain. In stretching, only the most intense feelings are heeded.

The precision necessary for each yoga pose is the guide to physical balance. The details of each pose are inexhaustible. For example, in any given standing pose the outer muscles of the leg work equally to those of the inner leg: the inside of the foot bears as much weight as the outside of the foot. The lower body may be supporting the torso, but the upper body is not passive. It is alive and complementing the alignment of the lower body. When doing yoga, attention is given to the front as well as to the back, to the sides, to the limbs, the joints, the musculation, the flow of energy, the breath.

But yoga can produce this physical balance only if the mind and body cooperate. This entails two elements: locating inner imbalances and then adjusting. While doing each pose the mind must be receptive to the messages the body is sending. Once the feelings are perceived, an adjustment may be made.

This intimate interplay between the body and mind is the essence of yoga. It is the main way in which yoga differs from mere stretching. To balance a pose it is simply impossible to let your mind wander to the grocery list, the house assessment, social entanglements, or the person next to you. Not that the mind doesn't do that, but when it does the balance of the pose dissipates and the mind must be pulled back "into" the body. To do yoga is similar to being a tightrope walker. A tightrope walker is never stationary, but is always moving because the balance on the rope is always changing. If he were to be totally still he would fall because balance is never to the right, never to the left, not always in the center. Balance is a continual readjustment and it requires incredible attention.

So yoga is very different from stretching. The degree of flexibility achieved does not determine success in yoga. Success is measured by a person's inward attention to the body and mind in the pose. Many times it is the less flexible students who do "real" yoga because the poses demand their attention. Flexible people sometimes find yoga elusive because their suppleness allows them to look as if they're doing yoga when really their attention is wandering.

3

Rationale and Results

Yoga exercises can benefit athletes in three major ways. In teaching an effective way to stretch and strengthen the body, yoga will promote physical balance, increase mental alertness, and help prevent injuries and discomforts. These changes, taken together, add up to greater bodily efficiency and result in improved athletic performance.

When you feel refreshed and attentive after exercise, it is because activity has stimulated the action of the muscles in pumping fluids through the body. More efficient pumping by the muscles depends on their level of elasticity; such elasticity will increase through the practice of yoga. In the same way, increased muscular flexibility and strength will prevent many common injuries and annoyances (muscle pulls, stiffness) that strenuous exercise can cause.

To understand how yogic stretching can accomplish these results, it is important to grasp certain facts about how our bodies function and move. The next few pages present this basic information and discuss the ways in which yoga can influence this functioning for better health and improved athletic performance.

THE PHYSIOLOGICAL CASE FOR STRETCHING

The power for athletic movement is produced by the contraction, or shortening, of muscles. Stretching can counteract the negative effects (spelled out below) of the repeated contractions which occur during running and other sports.

When you bend your forearm up, perhaps to show your muscles, it is the contraction of the biceps (upper arm muscles) that draws the arm up. To reverse the action of the arm in straightening the elbow, contraction of the opposing muscles, the triceps, must occur. During this latter contraction, the biceps lengthen, but only to accommodate the contraction of the triceps. The muscles act as a lever, and the joints as a fulcrum, when muscles contract. Movement is the result of muscles shortening; muscles pull bones together rather than pushing bones apart.

All athletic exertion, then, can be viewed as the repetitive and coordinated contraction of muscles and muscle groups. Such continual contractions determine the resting length of the *muscle spindle,* the "message center" of the muscle. When the spindle learns that the muscle is being asked continually to shorten, it adjusts to the demands placed upon it and becomes increasingly resistant to stretching or lengthening. Muscles that are persistently worked without stretching can thus become hard and short.

These bulging muscles conform to our traditional view of health and strength, but they are not pliable or adaptable. They deprive the body of optimum health by:

1. Inhibiting the movement of joints
2. Prohibiting full contraction of opposing or antagonist muscles
3. Misaligning the body
4. Causing general discomfort and inefficient movements
5. Increasing the possibility of injury, and
6. Deterring maximum pumping action within each muscle.

Inhibiting movement of joints. This potential difficulty is exemplified by what can happen to the muscles at the front of the groin. The huge amount of time we spend sitting — at the office, in our cars, in front of the television—causes the muscles that draw the thighs up to the torso to shorten, and they can no longer accommodate full movement in the hip socket. This joint is a ball in a socket, and is capable of a wide range of motion. But if the muscles at the front of the hip joint shorten, the leg is not able to move backward as far as it once could. The thigh bone is no longer being moved fully in the socket; this retards the flow of synovial fluid which lubricates the joints, and the chances of calcium build-up increase. Short muscles in the front of the groin also contribute to the common swayback condition when the front of the pelvis is pulled downward.

Prohibiting full contraction of opposing muscles. All muscles work in pairs. For example, as the muscles at the front of the groin draw the thigh up to the torso, the hamstring and buttock muscles lengthen. Conversely, to move the leg backwards the groin muscles lengthen as the hamstrings and buttocks shorten. But if the groin muscles are too tight they cannot lengthen fully, and their opposing muscles cannot contract completely. Muscles or portions of muscles that are not worked lose strength and tone, and they are less able to support and move the skeleton properly.

Misaligning the body. All muscles act as levers, and shortened muscles can pull the body out of alignment. This necessitates greater output of energy, and creates binds in the body which inhibit the flow of vital fluids.

Causing general discomfort. Stiffness of muscles and joints is often caused by muscles that are permanently shortened through strengthening without stretching, or by gross inactivity. This stiffness is a drain on the body's energy. For muscles to be semi-contracted in this way all the time, energy must be expended. Also, when a muscle is continually tight it cannot loosen to accommodate the contraction of its opposing muscle. This means that the brain, which receives the major portion of sensory information from muscles, is receiving confusing messages. When the brain receives a message to contract a muscle, the message is muddled if the opposing muscle is not lengthened. This leaves a person less efficient mentally.

Increasing chances for injury. A joint that is surrounded by tight, shortened muscles is structurally capable of tearing a muscle that cannot accommodate a given movement. If the muscle does not move freely, the joint may move without it, causing a dislocation, torn ligament, tendon, or muscle. Injury can also occur simply from chronic shortening. For example, if the hamstrings are continually shortened, as they are in running, they can compress the hip joint and/or knee joint. Such compression can lead to torn cartilage, pain in the hip, sciatica, or rotation at the knee.

Deterring maximum pumping action within muscles. Muscle action may be compared to a sponge. When the sponge is squeezed, equivalent to a muscle contracting, fluids flow. But for the sponge to absorb fluids efficiently again, it must be released and soft. So it is with muscles. If they are to pump efficiently they must be able to contract to move fluids onward, and then soften to absorb fluids they require.

These are dreary facts, but it is important that anyone who has embarked on a fitness plan be aware of them, and understand that there is a simple preventative solution: YOGA!

The basic purpose of the dynamic stretch, which is not used in yoga, (see p. 7) is to shorten a muscle. The simple knee-jerk reflex is a good example of this stretch. This reflex protects the muscles and surrounding joints from over-stretching when they have been stretched too far or too fast beyond their resting length.

The static stretch (see p. 7) involves positioning the body so that a muscle or muscle group is stretched, and then holding in this position. The static stretch lengthens the resting length of a muscle and thereby enhances resiliency. To bring about relaxation after sustained shortening activities, a muscle should be held in a sustained stretch position so that the cortex of the brain can first receive and then send out new "instructions" to the muscle spindle to lengthen.

Static stretching enhances our capacity for sensitivity to how we feel. Excessive muscular tightness means that the brain is always receiving messages from the stretch reflex system; such tightness makes the muscles very responsive to stretching, so that this reflex system is called upon to protect already shortened muscles. This continual stimulation of the brain makes it less sensitive to smaller messages from the body. By lengthening the resting length of muscles the stretch reflex is not elicited as often, permitting the brain to receive and respond to more subtle stimuli.

Static stretching also increases body strength. When you are stretching one muscle, its opposite muscle must be contracting. This muscle that is contracting has probably been weakened and has lost tone because it has been accommodating its antagonist muscle which is overly tight. Such weakening impairs the ability of the muscle to support the skeleton properly.

True strength, then, is more than just hardness. Pure strength is an important component of fitness—it provides stability and power. But flexibility is also crucial for adaptability. Genuine fitness means achieving balance between strength and flexibility.

For most people fitness is something over which we have power. By our chosen activities we can improve our health by doing more of what makes us feel better and less of what isn't beneficial. Although stretching is difficult at the outset, perseverance will be rewarded. All athletes, who are committed to a health-giving regimen, can benefit from the greater bodily strength and flexibility—in short, more complete and rounded fitness and health—which persistence in yoga will bring.

4

Getting Started

The information in this section deals with how you go about learning yoga. You may or may not have a teacher. If not, how do you select one? If you're not interested in a teacher or don't have access to one, how do you proceed on your own? How can this book be used to help you?

WITH OR WITHOUT A TEACHER

Yoga has traditionally been passed on from teacher to student. It is the best way to learn yoga. It is very difficult to see habitual imbalances embedded in your body and mind. These aberrations feel "normal." You aren't even aware of your unawareness. Teachers can often see what you can't. By offering the perspective of an interested outsider, the teacher can be a catalyst for increased awareness of your body.

If you are interested in a teacher try to find one who teaches in the Iyengar method (see Bibliography, p. 219). Find out if the person practices yoga regularly; the poses done while teaching class don't count. He or she should have information about correct movement and the leadership ability, courage and tact to enforce his or her judgment. Although you may find some trouble spots on your body you should feel generally better after two or three weeks in class. And of course, each teacher has his or her own style; find one who is appropriate to your likes, dislikes, and needs. If you have a teacher this book can reinforce the information and the numerous poses done in class.

If you choose not to work with a teacher it is possible to proceed on your own. The following information can serve as a guide to you.

YOGA ON YOUR OWN

When to do yoga. Regularity is the key to your yoga practice. Find some time in your day that you will have available regularly; maybe before or after your athletic workout, perhaps first thing in the morning. You should really practice six days out of seven, but if that seems excessive begin with every other day, or four days a week. You should not eat for two hours before practice.

Duration. In the beginning do yoga for ten to fifteen minutes at each practice. As your interest grows you will find that you naturally extend the time. For total balance you need to practice yoga equally as long as you do tightening activities.

Setting. Choose a clean, flat area where you can practice undisturbed. Do not work in direct sunlight. You will need a blanket or a mat.

Clothing. It is essential that you work with bare feet. Your shoes carry and reflect, and therefore reinforce, all the imbalances in your body. Wearing socks can lead to slippage and needless injury. Loose, comfortable clothing should be worn; your workout clothes are perfect.

Beginning a pose. First, meticulously follow the "placement" directions when entering each pose. This information is the basis for the balancing effects of yoga. If you walk with your feet turned out and stretch with your feet turned out you are reinforcing a misalignment. So pay close attention to the initial instructions. If the foundation is wrong the positive benefits of the pose are lost.

Move into the pose slowly. When movement is slow, it is more difficult to get hurt because your body gradually moves to its limit and there is no momentum to push it into injury. When movement is slow you can more easily feel which muscles are working and which part of your body needs attention.

Practical Suggestions for Your Beginning

1. If you have a special concern (e.g., abnormal blood pressure, a history of back pain or injury, pregnancy, or any physiological misalignment) please seek the advice of a qualified teacher before proceeding.

2. In the instructions the words in CAPITALS are essential for the safety of the pose; not all poses have these.

3. Select a clean room. Set aside a few minutes each day when you can practice undisturbed. Fifteen to twenty minutes a day is usually adequate in the beginning. When doing these poses outside, be sure you are on level ground, away from direct sunlight, and far from the "madding crowd." This gives you a chance to respond more carefully to how you feel.

4. Wait at least two hours after eating before beginning your practice. Evacuate your bladder and bowels before stretching.

5. Wear comfortable clothing that will allow your body to move. Always practice barefooted.

6. Breathe quietly through the nose. Most of the major movements should be done on an exhalation.

7. Soften the body and allow the brain to be alert and watchful. Keep eyes open at all times so you can check alignments and make adjustments. The use of a full length mirror can be very helpful.

8. Careful attention to your alignment is essential. Absorb the "placement" instructions for each pose.

9. Do not become dependent on the "aids." Work one day with them, the next day without them.

10. You will find you have a "good" side and a "bad" side. Occasionally do the bad side twice.

11. The poses you resist the most are likely the ones you need most.

12. Be persistent and energetic but at the same time be gentle and non-violent toward your Self.

Do not bounce. To bounce into a stretch activates the *dynamic stretch reflex,* the mechanism built into the muscles to prevent overstretching. To lengthen a muscle by bouncing or jerking makes it shorten automatically to protect itself from overstretching. So although a person stretching this way may say, "But I feel it stretch," in fact, he or she is actually tightening the muscles being worked on. It is an inefficient and incorrect way to stretch.

How far should you go into the pose? Go as far into the stretch as you can while maintaining the alignment described. It is much more beneficial to do the pose with correct alignment than to sacrifice the structure so that you appear to be stretching further.

You should be on the "edge" of your stretch, that is, feeling lots of sensation but not pain. If you are complacent changes will not occur; if you are overly ambitious you will get hurt.

Holding the pose. Once in the pose, hold it. In the beginning, poses should be held for ten to fifteen seconds. As your body gains flexibility and strength, slowly begin to increase the length of holds. Add five seconds at a time until you reach the maximum time described for each pose.

Attention. While holding the pose turn all your attention inward and consider: how do you feel? how does your body respond to the structure of the pose? where are you strong? where do you feel fatigue? where is the tightest spot? does the pose elicit any emotion? what do you learn about yourself? The possibilities are unending. Be receptive.

Breathe! Never hold your breath; it tightens the body. Always breathe through the nose with the mouth closed. Use your breath to stretch by moving on slow, steady, quiet exhalations. (Exceptions to this use of exhalations are noted in the illustrated descriptions.) Use the steady exhalation to give you a smooth and firm movement into and out of each pose.

Relaxation. In all phases of your practice, eliminate extra effort. Work the muscles necessary to hold the pose but notice and eliminate any tension in the eyes, face, neck, throat, shoulders, and stomach. These are the common areas where muscles are most frequently contracted. Then ferret out any other areas you are unnecessarily contracting. To do this you must consciously feel inwardly. There may be many spots like this. Once you have located the contracted areas, that information alone will enable you to release unnecessary muscular contractions.

Handling discomfort. While holding a pose, focus on the body area that has the most sensation. This is where the bind is. Many people deal with this type of discomfort by tightening the surrounding muscles in an attempt to protect the tight area. Instead, try the following response.

Get to know the binding area. Visualize what it might look like, how big it is, what shape it is. Has it a color? A personality? Does it moan, or does it fidget, jump, burn, or scream? Allow the bound area to increase; accept it. Relaxing or softening the binding area is the way to ease it and eventually eliminate it. Tightening muscles around the pain simply draws the bind more firmly into your body and you actually hang on to it.

What about pain? If you feel an uncontrollable pain, slowly leave the pose. Re-read the instructions. Adjust the pose to lessen the stretch (perhaps you will need to return to one of the earlier stages suggested with each pose.) Remember, overstretching is just as ineffective as understretching; neither has a place in a balanced yoga practice. Finally, seek the advice of a competent teacher if you are unable to respond properly to a persistent pain.

Adjusting poses. When you feel the need to change a pose, all changes should be made from the ground up. In standing poses, begin changes with the feet; in sitting poses, begin with the sitting bones and placement of the pelvis; in inverted poses, begin with the head, shoulders and elbows. Then, following the directions, work meticulously up from the ground. Never assume anything. Even though you may have placed your feet correctly, look at them and be sure. Make any necessary changes, then do the pose again.

Competition is out. Do not compete with yoga illustrations, your companion, your teacher, or yourself. Assess and accept your own stretching capacity. This capacity will change from day to day and from moment to moment. To be caught up in competition or athletic goals necessitates surrender of your inner awareness. When competition occurs in yoga, the joy of self-discovery remains elusive or simply disappears. Furthermore, on a very practical level, forcing a stretch in a competitive spirit can abuse or injure muscles, tendons, and ligaments. Work with your body and not with your ego.

Ending the pose. Care should be taken as you leave a pose. As you move out of the pose, focus on your alignment and breathe as slowly and evenly as you did when assuming the position originally. Reverse the directions given to do the pose, and in so doing, you contract the same muscles that were stretched. Sometimes you may "fall" or collapse out of a pose for one reason or another, but do not do this habitually. Abrupt posture changes will negate the strengthening that comes from proper movement and may also cause injury.

Working with imbalances. You will probably notice that one side of your body does not respond as quickly as the other. You may feel stiffer, weaker, or duller on this slow side. Sometimes it may be helpful to do a pose twice on your dull side since this side needs more care and attention than your more responsive side. Also, bring balance to your body and practice by reviewing the poses in the book frequently. If there are some poses you seldom or never do it may be a clue to the ones you need the most. Those poses are the ones you are likely to avoid.

Working with injuries.   Continue doing poses that do *not* affect the injured area. When you have an injury get permission of a physician before stretching the injured area. Take this book to the doctor and show him what you intend to do. In general, when you have injury to muscles, ligaments, or tendons do not stretch the area for three weeks. This gives it time to heal. Begin stretching the injured area by doing the easiest pose for that area. If the pose causes pain, discontinue for another week. If it does not cause pain, practice this one pose for two weeks. (It takes two to three weeks for a pose to affect the body.) If the area continues to improve after this time add another pose. Do these two poses for two weeks, then add a third, and so on. (If you add more than one pose at a time you will not know which pose is good or bad for the injury.) Proper movement can be therapeutic if you work intelligently. Working this way may seem slow. Acknowledge your impatience but know that methodical perseverance will pay off. If you are ambitious and push on you will have a constant reminder of your greed.

5

Digging In

The first section of this book gives you information *about* yoga. However, the rest of the book, the poses, form the most important section because they provide the framework within which you can derive benefits from yoga. The poses are most graphically illustrated by the pictures. The three models vary in flexibility, strength, and yoga experience. Using this combination of people shows how certain poses can be varied to meet different needs while working in the same general framework.

Don Nystrom runs 40 miles a week and has limited (10-1½ hour lessons) exposure to yoga. His poses show how you might look in the beginning. Tim Durbin played football in college, runs about 25 miles a week and has done yoga for a couple of years. Barbara Delisle is a yoga practitioner and teacher who runs.

The introduction to each section has important information on how to approach these particular poses. Some anatomical information is included to enhance your understanding of why it is best to move in a certain way. When a direction makes sense it will be easier to do what's being asked, and to remember correct movement and positioning. In the introduction there are also general directions for all of these poses to prevent undue repetitions. These may be the most important directions either for safety or for the effectiveness of the stretch. Please, read them.

Be sure to do the poses in the "Preliminaries" section first.

They seem simple, but are basic to the instructions given for all subsequent poses.

For organizational purposes the poses have been loosely categorized according to parts of the body. This is a false division because the body is a whole; while stretching the feet, the head is affected. Any forward bending pose stretches the entire back side, any backbending pose stretches the entire front side. So, you may find that the best pose for *you* to stretch *your* knee may be in the "hip" section. Bodies can vary so much that you simply must do a wide variety of poses to see what affects you the most. You have then become your best teacher.

Within each category the poses are given in the approximate order of difficulty. This is not always so because the degree of difficulty will depend on your body, and sometimes there is no way to determine which pose may be easier. No matter how flexible you think you are, do each successive pose until you find one that really "stretches" you, not "kills" you. Maybe one of the "easier" poses is exactly the one that will affect a certain "tight" spot. Practice this one.

Experience will quickly show you where you should be working. You will find discrepancies, e.g., you may be able to do the fifth hamstring stretch but only the first groin stretch. Follow your body's intelligence.

In the description of the poses the "placement" section is most important. It provides the foundation and can make the difference between a "stretch" and a "pose." It can make the difference between simply reinforcing misalignments and correcting them. Follow the directions and actual change will be manifested.

Usually, the completed "pose" follows the "placement." Many times you won't be able to do this pose, but it is shown so you can know the framework in which you are working. With the exception of the Shoulder Stand (see p. 156) and the Plough (see p. 158) I frequently teach a pose by having people "do" the completed pose first. This gives them information about their tightnesses and weaknesses. Also, this way they appreciate the aid or variation more. So you too may want to "do" the completed pose. If you can maintain the alignment of the pose then this is where you can work. However, do not dismiss the aids and/or variations. Often they can be the guide to deeper understanding of the poses.

If you can't maintain the alignment of the completed pose then you definitely need to examine the aids and variations. "Aids" illustrate the use of a prop to help you do the pose with proper alignment; sometimes they provide a lever for stretching, or protect parts of your body from over-stretching. Sometimes the aids are simply for balance. Whatever their purpose, do not think of them as demeaning. In the most "advanced" yoga classes props are used freely. I work with them in every practice.

"Variations" indicate that while doing the basic framework of the "pose" something is changed. Sometimes the intensity of the stretch is decreased, sometimes it is increased. If the effect is not stated it is because the accompanying photo shows the result. Even if you are working on the completed pose try the variations. It's guaranteed they'll teach you something new.

There are many poses in the book that are not classic yoga postures; for example, many of the hamstring stretches. They are included because they are necessary steps in preparing your body to do the poses. You can't do what you can't do, so there has to be a way to get there. Besides, by doing these poses with attention to how you feel, they become yoga. Doing anything with attention on how you feel becomes yoga.

One note concerning the names of the poses. The Sanskrit names given under the main heading for each pose are used internationally and are the original names. However, for convenience English substitutes are given. Sometimes the names are descriptive, sometimes they're a translation, as the fifth standing pose, Warrior II. It's really not important what you call them; it's important that you do them.

For your own yoga program you can proceed in one of two ways. Either follow the Practice Guide (see p. 205) or work progressively through corresponding poses (all first poses in each chapter, then all second poses, etc.) within each chapter. Either way it will probably take you six months to a year to do the more difficult poses. Once you are at that level, you can use the Core Program (see p. 209) as the basis of your regular practice.

The section on Areas of Concentration for Various Sports (p. 211) contains suggested poses for you to improve your performance and poses to counteract imbalances. The last group is important for injury prevention.

PART TWO
POSES

6

More Than Just Beginning: Preliminaries

The anatomical information and basic poses presented in this section are the foundation of all that follows; regardless of how flexible you may be, it's important that these fundamentals are understood at the outset.

The spine has four curves. The lower back and the neck are concave curves—they dip into the body. The tailbone area and rib cage are convex curves—they bulge out. For optimum health all four curves of the back should be preserved with no excessive compression or curving in any segment of the spine.

A long gentle S curve of the back insures proper spacing between the bones of the back, known as the vertebrae. Proper spacing of the vertebrae is important because nerves branch out from the spinal cord between the bones of the back. If the curves become more pronounced it means that there is compression on the inner side of the arch and the nerves that pass between those vertebrae suffer. The organs and structures enervated by these nerves decline.

In all movement, then, it is essential to preserve and nurture the four gentle curves of the back. *The placement of the pelvis determines the curves of the back.* Therefore, before you begin stretching it is important that you get in touch with the muscles that move the pelvis.

Here are two ways to practice tilting the pelvis. When practicing these poses be attentive to the lower back. Note how the alternate positions of the pelvis reverse the arch of the lower back.

PELVIC TILTING ON HANDS AND KNEES

1. Placement: Make yourself into a table. Place the knees three to four inches apart, under the center of the hip sockets. Place the hands ten or twelve inches apart, under the center of the shoulder sockets. The middle fingers point straight ahead. The thighs and arms are parallel and far enough apart to enable the back to be flat.

2. Cat tilt. On an exhalation, contract the buttocks and tuck your tailbone down, drop the head, and allow the back to hump up like an angry cat.

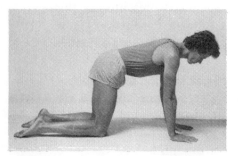 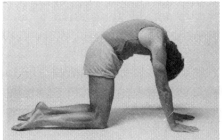

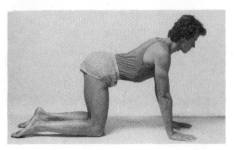

Clockwise From Left: Pelvic Tilting-Placement; Cat Tilt; Dog Tilt

3. Dog tilt. On an inhalation, lift the sitting bones, look forward *not* up, open chest toward chin and allow the back to arch slightly, like a dog stretches after a nap.

PELVIC TILTING LYING ON YOUR BACK

1. Placement: Lie on your back, bend the knees and place the feet in front of the sitting bones, six to eight inches from the body. Roll the upper edge of the shoulders back toward the ground, open the chest. Arms are extended next to the body, palms down.

2. Cat tilt. Squeeze the buttock muscles and lift the tailbone slightly off the floor. The lower back flattens into the floor. At first you will have to tighten your stomach to do this. Later, practice with the belly soft and relaxed. This is important for correct posture. Eventually, when standing, the pelvis is tucked and the stomach relaxed. (A contracted abdomen pulls the rib cage down and compresses the lungs.)

3. Dog tilt. Contract the muscles of the back and lift the waist off the floor. The front of the body lengthens. Do not press the back of the head into the floor. The arms stretch down toward the feet. The hands and arms are active but not tense.

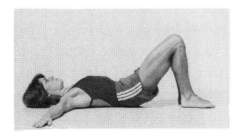

Cat Tilt

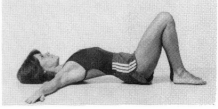

Dog Tilt

As you can see, even though the general position of the body has changed, the pelvic tilt is the same regardless of whether you start on your back or on hands and knees. Because the pelvic tilt is so important in all further instructions it will facilitate communication to name the alternate positions of the pelvis. When the tailbone is tucked down, the pelvic position will be called the "cat tilt;" when the sitting bones are lifted the pelvic position will be called the "dog tilt." In general, the cat tilt is used in all standing and back-bending positions. The dog tilt is used in all forward-bending poses.

Besides using these movements to get in touch with the pelvis they are also an excellent way to relieve tension built up in the lower back. Gently reverse from cat tilt to dog tilt in the pose you find most effective.

LIFTING THE KNEECAPS

The knee joint is frequently called the "holy joint" because it should be treated with respect and care. Not only is it very complex because of crossing ligaments and vulnerable cartilage, but it also supports weight. To strengthen and protect the knees the quadriceps (thigh muscles) must be contracted when stretching the legs. Practice the following:

1. Placement. Stand erect, feet comfortably apart. Bend over and place your thumbs above your kneecaps, fingers wrapped around the back of the knees. The legs must be straight.

2. Pose. Contract the thigh muscles, the quadriceps, and draw the kneecaps up. Feel how the thumbs rise. Do this often in the beginning. Once you get the feel of it you no longer need to place the thumbs above the knees.

For any pose in which one or both of the legs is straight the knee is contracted in this manner. The instruction frequently is,

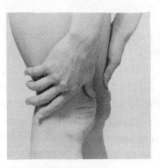

Lifting The Knee Caps-
Placement

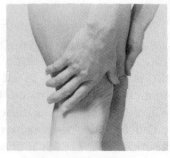

Pose-Tightened Knees

"Pull the kneecap up," or, "Tighten the knee." Always think of the kneecap lifting up, *not going back.*

SQUARING THE FEET

Most people are tighter on the inner edges of their feet and legs than on the outer edges. To find out whether you are in this group, stand in a neutral position with the feet parallel and flat on the floor. If your knees turn in toward the mid-line of the body you have this inner leg tightness. When lining the knees up over the feet the inner edges of the feet lift off the floor.

This means that when you walk and run, you probably land with more weight on the outside of the feet, legs, knees, and hips before the weight slides to the inner edge. This can lead to over-use injuries and/or over-mobility in the bones of the foot which then must be compensated for by the entire body.

The best single pose to alleviate this imbalance is the Hero's Pose (see p. 87) and all of its variations. *In all other poses keep the feet squared.* To learn this do the following.

1. Sit sideways to a wall. Lie on your back and straighten your legs up the wall. Turn your feet so the soles are parallel to the ceiling. (If your legs bend, move 2 or 3 inches away from the wall, or until you're comfortable.) The joints under your big toes should touch, the heels are slightly apart.

Your feet will probably look like the picture, with the inner edges of the feet drawn down toward the body, the outer edges up toward the ceiling.

To square the feet press the inner edges of the feet up and draw back the outer edges until the soles of the feet are "flat," square to the ceiling.

2. Another way to practice squaring the feet is to sit on the floor with feet pressing evenly into a wall. Keep legs straight with kneecaps tight. You can lean back on your hands.

3. When standing, feel pressure on the ball joints under your big toes. Press here but lift the arches of the feet. To line the knees up with the feet, contract the buttocks and roll both legs outward,

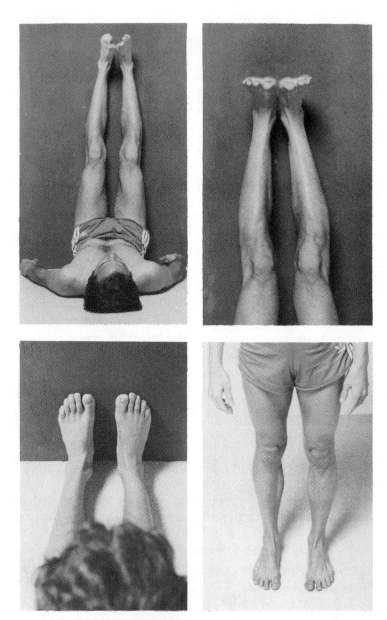

From Top Left: Unaligned Feet; Properly Squared Feet; Seated-
Feet Squared Against a Wall; Standing-Feet Squared

away from the midline of the body. To accomplish this with the feet flat will take TIME!!!

Squaring your feet will be easiest to do when you can see them, as in the sitting poses. Become familiar with how it *feels* so you can apply it in all the poses, even when lying down, backbending and so on.

7

Self-Reliance:
The Standing Poses

The standing poses are extremely important for minimizing the curves of the back as well as elongating and strengthening the spine. No matter what these poses require, always position the pelvis so that your back has four gentle curves. The instructions will help you to do this, but some people may have to modify them slightly according to the needs of their backs. Maintaining length in the back during these poses strengthens muscles that support proper posture.

Standing postures also stretch and strengthen the legs. For athletes, learning these poses will improve posture and increase fluidity in the joints of the lower body.

All standing poses begin in the Mountain Pose (see p. 35), even if the final pose is done with the legs apart. Starting in the Mountain Pose assures proper alignment. To get from the Mountain Pose to a split-leg stance requires a jump. This jump provides better balance than just stepping from one foot to the other.

Jumping. To learn the correct jump, stand in Mountain Pose. Inhale as you bend both knees, and bring elbows to shoulder level with middle fingers almost touching. Even though the arms move toward the center line of the body, don't collapse the chest. Exhale and jump the feet apart to the spread desired for each pose. The jump should be low and silent, so land on the balls of the feet, descend to the heels with control. The feet should still be parallel and even, that is, the toes should touch an imaginary line drawn from foot to foot. As the legs split, the arms extend straight out, from the shoulders, inner elbows up, palms down.

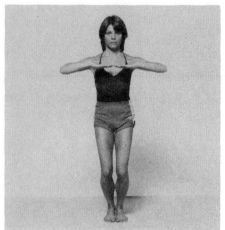

Preparation For Jumping

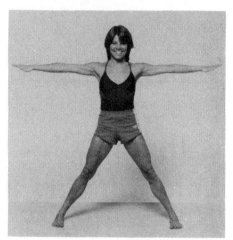

Completed Jump

Turning the feet. Many poses then instruct you to turn one foot out and one foot in. The reference point for this direction is the midline of the body. The heel of the foot that turns out (usually called the front foot) should be opposite the arch of the foot that turns in (called the back foot). See illustration.

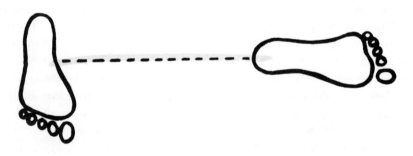

Back Foot   Front Foot

Weighting the feet. When doing the standing poses ideally the weight on each foot should be balanced in the center of the foot. You will soon learn how difficult this is. To bring balance to the feet while doing any split leg pose with the feet turned, *put more weight on the inside of the forward foot and more weight on the outside of the back foot.*

Protecting the knees. To avoid twisting the knees lift the knee-caps first then turn the feet. Keep the knees tight throughout the pose. Always keep the knees directly in line with the feet, even if one hip must move forward. To avoid overextending the knees (arching back too far) tuck the pelvis firmly in cat tilt; lift knee-caps high, *not* back.

Caution: If you have problem knees proceed as follows: First do leg lifts with working leg straight, i.e., kneecap tight, other leg bent, foot on floor. Also, sit on table with thighs stabilized, lower legs hanging. Straighten one leg at a time, tighten kneecap and hold 5 to 10 seconds. Alternate 10 times (daily for 2 to 4 weeks.) Next add standing poses with legs straight, e.g., Triangle Pose. (4 times a week for 2 to 4 months.) Then move on to standing poses with one or both knees bent. Finally proceed to Thigh Strength-ener (see p. 104), beginning with 20 second holds, and increasing the time five seconds a week until you can hold 2 to 4 minutes.

MOUNTAIN POSE

(Tadasana)

1. Placement. Stand with legs straight, feet together, big toes touching and in line. Line knees up so they face directly forward. Hips, shoulders, and eyes should be level and facing forward. Chin is parallel to floor.

2. Pose. Tighten the thighs and lift the kneecaps. Tighten the buttocks, tucking the tail under (cat tilt). Lift the sternum (breast bone) toward the ceiling. Chin level, throat loose. The shoulders roll down and back, arms remain loose.

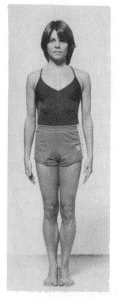
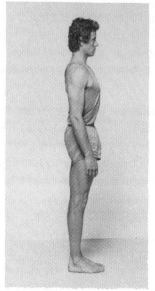
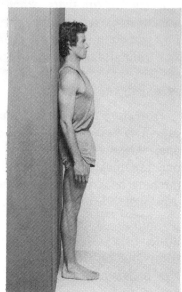

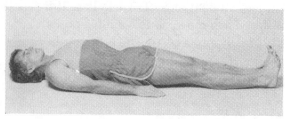

Clockwise From Top Left:
Mountain Pose-Placement;
Mountain Pose-Side View;
Mountain Pose Against Wall;
Mountain Pose on Floor

3. Variation. Bisect the front of your body with an imaginary line. See if the weight is evenly distributed on both sides. Examine the response of the right foot, then the left. Observe in this manner (with the entire body) as you move up the center line. See if elongating the dull parts helps give the pose an "alive" feeling.

4. Aid. Heels close to wall, tuck buttocks, touch head and flatten shoulder blades to wall. Using same centering line, see if both sides of body touch, respond to the wall in exactly the same way.

5. Aid. Lie on back with torso in straight line, face directly up. Bend knees and place feet on floor. Do cat tilt, open chest, move shoulder blades and shoulders gently away from ears. Palms down, stretch fingers. Slowly move the feet out until the legs are straight with kneecaps pulled up. Feet vertical and squared toes together, heels one inch apart. With neck and face soft, lengthen the spine.

6. Aid. Do this pose facing a full length mirror. What muscles do you have to activate to lift arches, get the knees straight, tailbone down, and collar bones horizontal? When lifting the chest be sure it rises and does *not* move forward. Here you should see where you are asymmetrical. You need to stretch the compressed areas.

7. Variation. People with knock knees will not be able to get their feet together unless they cross their knees. In this case it is better to have the inner edges of the knees together and the feet apart but parallel.

Benefits: realigns body, stretches legs, opens chest, steadies the breath, forms foundation for all other poses.

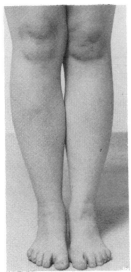
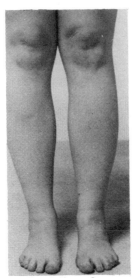

Knock Knees-Incorrect
Placement of Feet

Knock Knees-Correct
Placement of Feet

STANDING SIDE STRETCH

1. Placement. From Mountain Pose place the feet twelve inches apart, and parallel. Inhale and bring the arms straight up alongside the ears. Interlock the fingers.

2. Pose. Exhale, push the palms toward the ceiling. With the exception of the arms, the body is in Mountain Pose, so the buttocks and legs are firm. Hold for a few breaths, release and change the finger position (different leading thumb). Repeat, gradually increasing time.

3. Variation. From No. 2, take the torso to the right for a few breaths and then to the left. Keep the legs straight. Release and change the interlock; repeat.

4. Aid. Hold a tie or belt between your hands. In this way the arms can stretch up while the shoulders move down and away from the ears. If you cannot straighten your elbows with your hands clasped overhead, be sure to work with this aid.

Benefits: Good stretch given to both sides of waist and hips. Shoulders and arms strengthened.

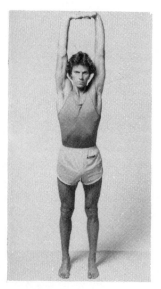
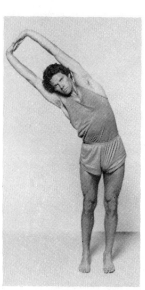
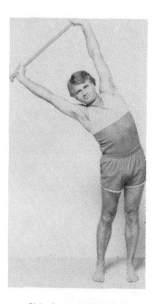

Standing Side Stretch-Pose   Side Stretch Variation   Side Stretch With Belt

TREE POSE

(Vrksasana I)

1. Placement. Stand in Mountain Pose. Exhale, bend right knee up and hold right inner ankle with right hand, place right foot as high as possible on left inner thigh. Left leg in Tadasana position, *pelvis in cat tilt. Align pelvic bones and hips with shoulders.* To do this the knee may come in toward the center.

2. Pose. Palms press together in "namaste," chest stays open as in Tadasana. Eventually knee moves to side as hips and groins become looser. Foot and thigh press firmly together, weight on *inner* and outer edge of the left foot. Chin parallel to floor, throat and eyes soft. Hold 15 to 20 seconds, release and reverse.

3. Variation. Stretch arms up, keep shoulders down. If right hip still goes back too far with right knee in toward center, then lower right foot on thigh. *Do not bend left leg.*

4. Aid. Stand against wall if balance is difficult. Tuck buttocks under, place hands on hips to judge whether hips are level.

Benefits: Loosens hips, groins, opens chest. Checks and steadies the nerves.

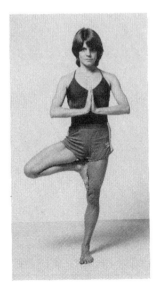
Tree Pose

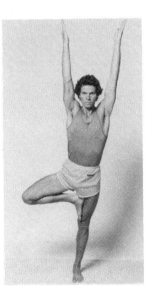
Arms Lifted in Tree Pose

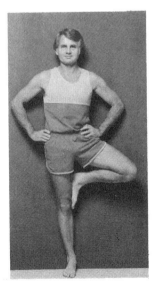
Back Against Wall

TRIANGLE POSE

(Trikonasana)

1. Placement. Begin in Mountain Pose, jump feet apart approximately 3 to 3½ feet (or length of one of your legs). Turn left foot in 30 degrees, right foot out 90 degrees. *Right heel points toward middle of back foot. Align right knee with right foot. Kneecaps up.*

2. Pose. Exhale, move hips toward the left, maintaining cat tilt. *Bend at the hips, not the waist.* Extend entire torso sideways and out along right leg, not forward and down. Extend right arm downwards without disturbing the rest of the pose. Stretch left arm vertically. Turn head to see left thumb. Hold 15 to 20 seconds. Release by coming back to center and reverse.

3. Variation. Place right hand in right groin, push right hand toward left hip on exhalation. Place right hand on right thigh, shoulders down. Head faces straight. Press the weight on the ball of the right foot and the outer edge of left foot.

4. Aid. Place right heel against wall with left foot turned out at 90 degree angle. Do pose as in No. 2. Wall helps keep right leg straight and right heel down.

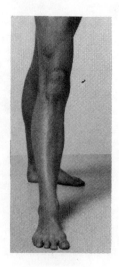
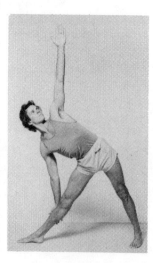
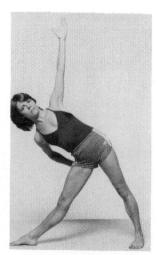

Triangle Pose-
Foot Placement

Triangle Pose

Triangle Pose-Hand in Groin

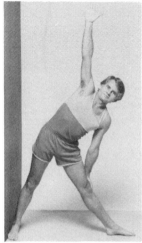

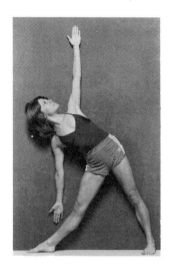

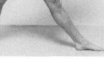

Heel Against Wall

Triangle Pose-Back Against Wall

5. Aid. The wall can help you to keep the body lateral in this pose. Stand with your back against a wall; the left heel touches the wall, the right foot is opposite the left arch and parallel to the wall. Proceed as in No. 2 or 3. Work to keep the left hip and shoulder blade on the wall. Place more weight on the outside of the left foot and on the inside of the right foot. Reverse.

Benefits: Stretches and strengthens feet, ankles, and knees. Frees hips and chest, elongates spine.

WARRIOR POSE II

(Virabhadrasana II)

1. Placement. Stand in Mountain Pose. Jump 4 to 4½ feet apart, extend arms from shoulder. Turn left foot in 30 degrees, right foot out 90 degrees. Align feet as in Triangle Pose.

2. Pose. Exhale, maintain body in Mountain Pose as you bend right knee to form a right angle. *Keep the perpendicular imaginary line down the front of the body.* Take left shoulder back slightly to open chest. Tuck buttocks under, keep the left groin moving back and slightly downwards. The back leg should be straight.

3. Variation. Beginners may not be taking the bent leg to a right angle, but they must keep the knee in line with the heel, forming a perpendicular lower leg. You may keep hands on waist. Back heel down.

4. Aid. Stand with back to wall, in position No. 1. Left heel should touch wall. Move into the pose (No. 2). Use the wall to help you maintain your Tadasana awareness, keeping arms, shoulder blades, and buttocks to wall. *Right knee moves exactly in line with foot, staying parallel with wall. The left hip may come forward. For safety it is more important to align the knee with the foot than to keep the left buttock on the wall.*

Benefits: Develops stamina, intense stretch given to groins. Strengthens the back and the legs.

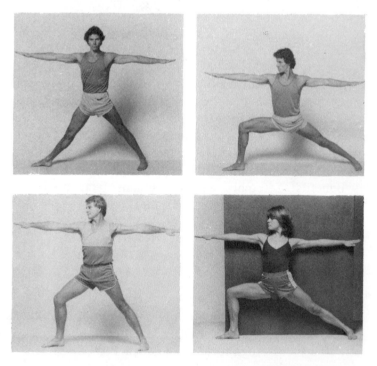

Left to Right From Top: Warrior Pose II-Placement; Completed Warrior Pose II; Warrior Pose II-Short Stance; Warrior Pose II-Back Against Wall

EXTENDED LATERAL POSE

(Parsvakonasana)

1. Placement. From Mountain Pose, jump 4 to 4½ feet apart, arms extended horizontally, palms down. Turn left foot in 30 degrees, right foot out 90 degrees. Align feet as in Triangle Pose.

2. Pose. On exhalation, *bend right knee in line with right foot, with outer edge of knee pointing to little toe.* Exhale, stretch right side of body from right hip, extending along right thigh. With the right hand, fingertips or palm, on floor, straighten left arm over left ear. Turn from hips to face the ceiling. Hold 10 to 20 seconds, reverse.

3. Variation. Taking the knee to a right angle is difficult in the beginning, so narrow the stance to 3½ feet then bend the right leg so that the *lower leg is perpendicular* to the floor. Hold the inside of the right lower leg with the right hand. Press the left arm against the leg and open the chest. Keep back leg strong and straight.

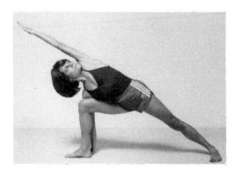

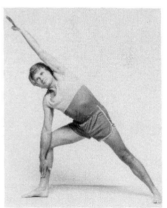

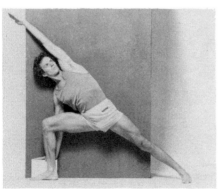

Clockwise From Top Left: Extended Lateral Pose; Extended Lateral Pose-Short Stance; Back Against Wall in Extended Pose

4. Aid. Place the left heel against a wall, feet placed as in No. 1. Place two thick books behind your right foot. Do the pose as in No. 2, placing the right palm on the books (use the fingertips and/or more books if you are working in thigh/knee position No. 3.)

Benefits: Intense stretch given to both legs, sides of body. Opens and loosens the hips, groins.

INTENSE SIDE STRETCH

(Parsvottanasana)

1. Placement. Standing in Mountain Pose, press the palms together in back, fingers pointed up, forming "namaste." *Do not do "namaste" with the concave chest, instead see No. 3.* Jump 3 to 3½ feet apart, take left foot in 80 degrees, right foot out 90 degrees. Turn the entire body to face right. *Lift the kneecaps.*

2. Pose. Inhale with the pelvis in cat tilt, open the chest by stretching slightly back from the hips. Exhale, extend the torso forward from the hips, pelvis in dog tilt. Stretch the left side a little more to allow the right hip to go back, the left hip to move forward. Place chin on shin. *Keep both legs straight,* back heel down.

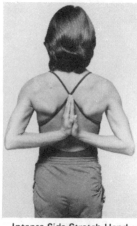

Intense Side Stretch-Hand Position

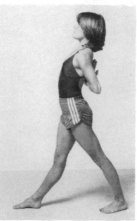

Placement-Intense Side Stretch

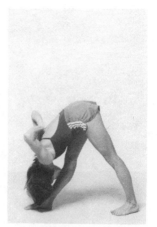

Intense Side Stretch

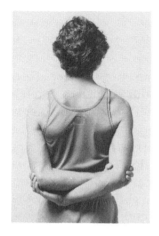
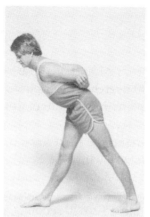
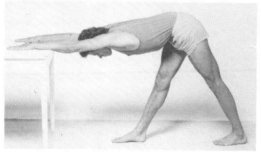

Clockwise From Top Left: Hand Variation-Intense Side Stretch; Variation of Pose; Hands Supported in Intense Side Stretch

3. Variation. Bend the elbows, holding the elbows, forearms or the wrists if: "namaste" is impossible, or if your upper back is concave with shoulders rounded in order for you to do "namaste." Do No. 2, taking the sternum forward and not down, keeping the back flat. In the beginning, extend out without taking the chin down.

4. Aid. Facing a ledge that is approximately waist level, stand an arm's length away. Do No. 2, extending the hands to the ledge, pressing the wrists, extending the fingers to lift and lengthen the spine, centering the sternum above the right thigh. Continue stretching toward the ledge, walking the fingers forward *without shifting the weight off the back foot. Create the dog tilt with the pelvis.*

WARRIOR POSE I

(Virabhadrasana I)

1. Placement. From Mountain Pose, jump 4 to 4½ feet apart. Turn left foot in 80 degrees, turn right foot out 90 degrees. Stretch arms straight up, palms in, shoulders down. The entire body faces right.

2. Pose. Exhale, bend the right knee to form a right angle, keeping the left leg straight with left heel on floor. Tuck the pelvis firmly down in cat tilt. *Extend the body up as you bend the knee. Bent knee stays in line with heel.* Look up slightly. Eventually the hands are joined. Hold 15 to 20 seconds, reverse.

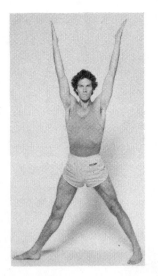 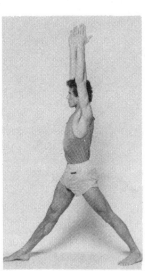 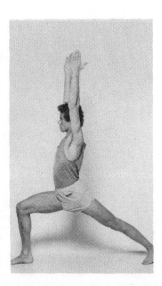

Warrior Pose I-Placement   Torso Turned-Warrior Pose I   Warrior Pose I

3. Variation. If forming a right angle is extremely difficult, then narrow the stance and focus on maintaining the shin of the right leg perpendicular. Stretch the arms out horizontally if taking them up vertically also raises the shoulders near ears. Keep the gaze straight ahead, chin parallel to floor.

4. Aid. Keep the back heel against a wall, turn toes under, square hips. Push the heel against wall to keep back leg straight.

Benefits: Excellent for opening the chest and for strengthening the shoulders and arms. Also strengthens knees and stretches ankles and calves.

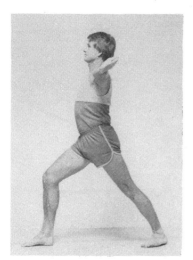
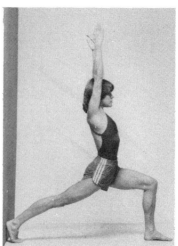

Short Stance-Warrior Pose I   Heel Against Wall in Warrior Pose I

REVOLVED TRIANGLE

(Parivrtta Trikonasana)

1. Placement. From Mountain Pose, jump 3 to 3½ feet apart. Turn left foot in 60 degrees, right foot out 90 degrees. *Take care to align feet properly; keep kneecaps tight.* The arms are extended from the shoulders.

2. Pose. Exhale, swing the entire left side around to the right. Bend from the hips and place left hand on the floor parallel and near to the outer edge of the right foot. Keep the left heel on the floor. The arms and shoulders stretch away from the chest to form a single vertical line. Turn head to look at right thumb. Extend the spine horizontally. Hold 15 to 20 seconds, come up from the hips, reverse.

3. Variation. Do No. 1. Take the right hand to the right groin. Bend the left arm making a fist with the left hand, lift the left elbow and, with an upward movement, swing the left elbow around to the right. This gives you the feeling of the movement that takes you into the pose. Repeat several times and reverse.

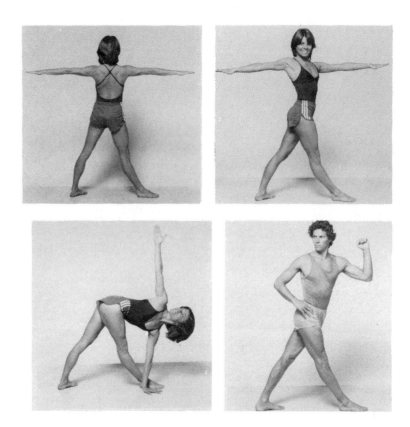

Left to Right, From Top: Revolved Triangle-Placement; Torso Turned-Revolved Triangle; Completed Pose; Torso Rotation in Revolved Triangle

4. Aid. Stand in No. 1, back to wall and six inches away. Place two books between wall and right foot. Exhale, swing torso to right to face wall, bend arms and walk fingers as far to right as possible. Turn head to right. Body leans toward right hand, legs remain straight. Keeping right elbow and hand on wall, bend from hips to left and elongate chest and back. Take the left fingertips down to books (right forearm will slide across wall). Lift buttocks in dog tilt. Straighten both arms, right arm and left ear on wall. Eventually do this with both elbows and hands on wall as you move to left. Reverse.

5. Aid. Begin as in No. 1. Place a chair so legs of chair straddle your right foot. Exhale, turn to right so you face the chair. Square the body. Step solidly on left heel, bend at the hips and place fingertips on chair seat. If the bones at the back of your waist poke out, place hands on back of chair and straighten arms. With chin slightly in, work to elongate spine; right side should be as long as left side.

Caution: If knee pains occur, try taking the back heel up and pivoting on the ball of the back foot. If pain persists discontinue until a teacher is consulted.

Benefits: Good for lower back discomfort, especially after backward bending poses. Strengthens and stretches the legs and increases flexibility in the hips.

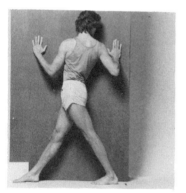

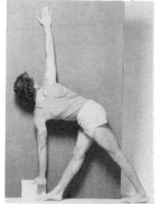

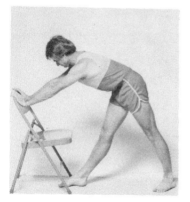

Clockwise From Top Left: Preliminary Revolved Triangle with Wall; Completed Revolved Triangle; Revolved Triangle-Working with Chair

HALF MOON POSE

(Ardha Chandrasana)

1. Placement. Do Triangle Pose (see p. 40). Bend right knee, placing right fingers on floor one foot ahead and a little behind right foot. Place left arm along body.

2. Pose. Exhale, shift weight forward to right leg. Lift straight left leg as right leg straightens to carry body. Tuck the right buttock under firmly and *open the left hip to the ceiling.* Left shin parallel to floor, push left foot away. Extend left arm straight up, turn head as in Triangle Pose. Hold 10 to 15 seconds, exhale back to Triangle Pose, reverse.

3. Variation. Do No. 2, but keep left arm along body, head facing forward. Bring the right lung forward, softening the right waist. Work high up on right fingertips.

4. Aid. Place two books along wall. Stand with back to wall so that your left (balancing) hand will be on books. Do No. 2, keeping left fingertips on books. Tuck left buttocks under and revolve right buttock back to touch wall. Right heel, shoulder, wrist also touch wall.

Benefits: Excellent for loosening the groins and hips. Strengthens the ankle, lengthens and creates flexibility in the spine. Aids in developing a sense of balance in the body.

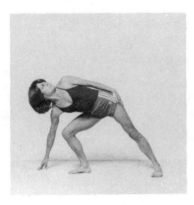

Half Moon Pose-Placement

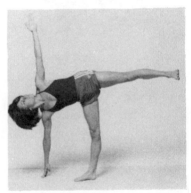

Half Moon Pose

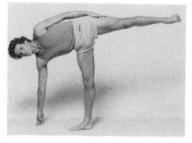

Arm Variation-Half Moon Pose

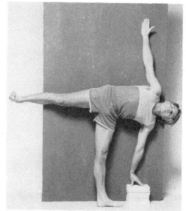

Back Against Wall-Half Moon Pose

WARRIOR III

(Virabhadrasana III)

1. Placement. Do Warrior I (see p. 46) to the left. Exhale, extend the torso along the left thigh, stretching the trunk forward from the hips. Rest the torso lightly on the thigh.

2. Pose. Exhale, straighten the left leg while lifting the right leg. The right leg remains straight and in line with the arms. The buttocks are level; if necessary, drop the right side to align the body. Body forms a "table" with the left leg perpendicular and the right leg, torso, and arms parallel to the floor. The torso moves forward, the right leg stretches backward. Press the right heel out. Hold for several breaths, gradually increasing to 20 seconds. Return to Warrior I, reverse.

3. Variation. Begin in Warrior I with the arms extended to the sides or stretched up without joining the palms. Maintain either arm position as you do the balance. Keep the gaze straight ahead and never down.

4. Aid. Use either a wall or a ledge to support the hands as you balance and keep the buttocks level.

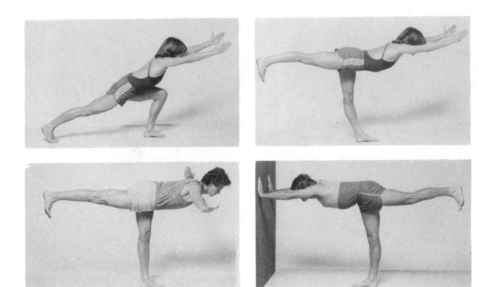

Left to Right From Top: Warrior III-Placement; Warrior III pose; Arm Variation-Warrior III; Hands on Wall-Warrior III

Benefits: Enables one to feel the dynamic qualities inherent in balance. Especially recommended for runners.

EXTENDED TOE TO HAND POSE

(Utthita Hasta Padangusthasana)

1. Placement. Stand in Mountain Pose. Shift weight to right leg, bend left knee and lift left thigh to chest. Hold left big toe between thumb and next two fingers. Right hand on right hip.

2. Pose: Exhale, straighten the left leg, kneecap tight. Keep hips and shoulders level. Pull leg higher and hold with both hands. Hold 10 to 15 seconds. Increase to 30 seconds then to 1 minute. Reverse.

3. Aid. Stand in Mountain Pose facing a ledge, the seat of chair, any table or desk, sink, etc. Place right heel or ankle on ledge, push heel out until foot is vertical. Place hands on hips. When reversing be sure to hold equal amount of time.

4. Aid. To aid balance hold back of chair or any ledge, even a wall.

Benefits: Stretches and strengthens legs, increases balance.

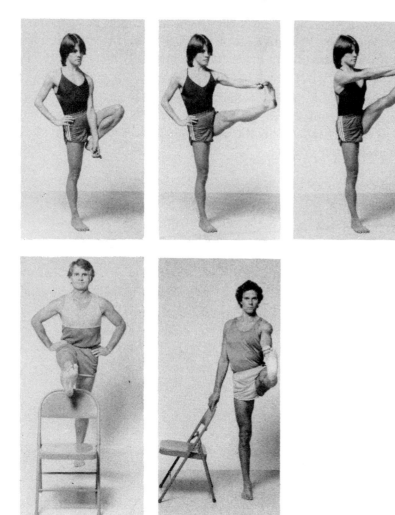

Left to Right From Top: Extended Toe to Hand Pose-Placement; Extended Toe to Hand Pose With One Hand; Using Two Hands; With Foot Supported; Balance Aid Used in Pose

SITTING ON NOTHING AT ALL

(Utkatasana)

1. Placement.   Stand in the Mountain Pose. Stretch the arms straight up, turn the palms so they face each other.

2. Pose: Exhale, squat until the thighs are parallel to the floor. Do not lean over the knees, keep the back as vertical as possible. Hold for a few breaths in the beginning, gradually increasing to 20 to 30 seconds. Release back to Mountain Pose.

3. Variation. Do the pose with the feet slightly apart and stretch the arms horizontally to aid your balance. Eventually take the arms to the vertical, closing the palms only if the shoulder can stay down away from the ears.

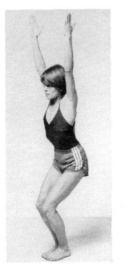
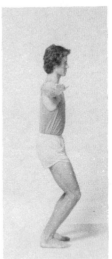
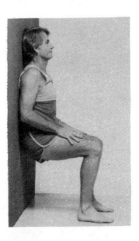

Back Against Wall

Sitting on Nothing-Pose   Arm and Foot Variation

4. Aid. Do this pose with the back completely against a wall, feet apart in line with the hips. Put arms up or hands on thighs. If the legs are very weak, sit on the edge of a chair and do the pose with the arms stretching upward.

Benefits: Strengthens the thighs and ankles. Opens the chest.

Continual practice of the standing poses can not be over-emphasized. They prepare the body for all other poses by developing spinal elongation and building overall strength of the body. They also bring flexibility to the legs. An excellent way for a beginner to proceed would be to spend the first six months to a year focusing mainly on the poses in this chapter. To round out your beginning practice do a variation of the Hero's Pose (p. 87), the Shoulder Stand (p. 156) , and the Corpse Pose (p. 200).

8

Save the Psoas:
Stomach Strengtheners

Leg lifts strengthen the stomach and the lower back. But as anyone with a bad back knows, if these are done incorrectly, or before the body is strong enough, leg lifts can cause painful backaches. Here's why.

Attached to the *front side* of the lumbar spine (the waist or lower back area) is the psoas muscle, a very important muscle for overall posture. It attaches to the belly side of all five lumbar vertebrae, then descends downward in the pelvis, crosses the hip joint, and connects to the inner edge of the thigh bone. This muscle initiates walking; it lifts the thigh bone up.

The muscles that act in opposition to the psoas are the abdominals, the muscles that line the surface of the stomach or lap area. For correct positioning of the pelvis the psoas and abdominals should have equal tone, flexibility and strength. One example of imbalance between these sets of muscles is the sway back. As shown in the illustration, in this imbalance the abdominal muscles are lax, so the psoas has to overwork to hold the body upright. The psoas, held in a state of semi-contraction, then shortens. This pulls the lower back forward, overarching the spine and compressing the discs of the lower back. This spells misery!

You can see why runners may be prone to this type of muscular imbalance. Running tightens the outer back muscles and repeatedly

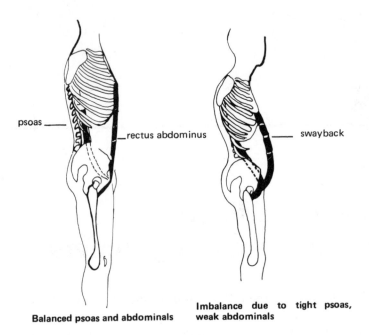

psoas

rectus abdominus

swayback

Balanced psoas and abdominals

Imbalance due to tight psoas, weak abdominals

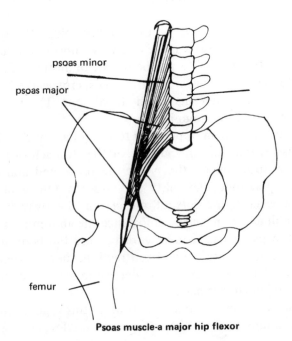

psoas minor

psoas major

femur

Psoas muscle-a major hip flexor

contracts the psoas to lift the legs with each stride. Muscles connected to the back work much more than the stomach muscles. So unless one works to strengthen the stomach area, running promotes a basic structural imbalance characterized by a tight back and psoas and a weak belly.

Leg lifts can strengthen the stomach if done correctly. They can strain the back if done incorrectly. *Always tuck the pelvis into the cat tilt* (see p. 28) *and keep the lower back on the floor throughout the poses.* If the back comes up it means the legs are being lifted by the psoas, a back muscle. To activate the stomach and reinforce the back, keep the lower back long, on the floor. Working any other way reinforces an imbalance and may be dangerous.

Unless you are in top physical shape or working with a teacher, don't do the full body sit-ups that used to be taught in school. The rationale for sit-ups is to strengthen the stomach. However, when doing traditional sit-ups the muscles that flex the hip do the major part of the work.

The stomach muscles can flex the torso about 30 degrees; to lift higher into a full sit-up the hip flexors must be contracted. This may strain the psoas muscle. It is designed to lift the thigh bone, but not the torso which is much heavier. This is why sit-ups can cause back strain.

Instead of the classical sit-ups use the variations given here. As in leg lifts, always *keep the lower back on the floor.*

When you can do leg lifts and sit-ups with no strain, and you understand how to protect your back, then begin practicing the Boat Pose. (see p. 63)

LEG LIFTS

1. Placement. Lie on the back with the entire body on a straight line, a reclining Mountain Pose. Turn the feet as shown, keep feet squared. *Tuck pelvis in cat tilt.* Open the chest, lower shoulders, palms down. Relax neck and throat. If your chin is above your forehead in this position, place something under the head so your face is parallel to the floor.

2. Variation. Bend both knees, feet parallel near buttocks. Bend left knee over chest. Exhale, press lower back to floor, push left heel away, kneecap up. Exhale, lower leg to floor with control. Build to 10 repetitions with each leg. Reverse procedure by dragging heel on floor until leg is straight; lift leg to vertical, bend knee over chest, place foot on floor. Build to 10 repetitions.

3. Variation. Do. No. 2 above except straighten the leg on the floor. Pay attention not to push off with this leg or the back of the head. When lifting both legs, bend knees over chest, exhale, press waist to floor and lower legs. Don't lift straightened legs together yet.

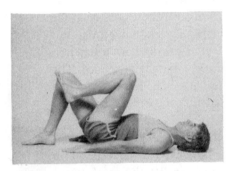
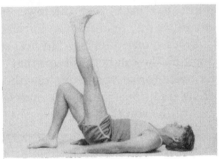
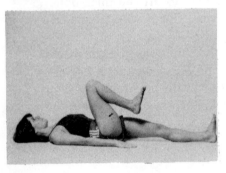

Clockwise From Top Left: Leg Lifts-Both Knees Bent; Working Leg Straightened; Non-Working Leg Straight

4. Variation. When you can do the above comfortably keep both legs straight all the time (see picture below). Begin in No. 1. Exhale, press the lower back down and lift one leg to 90 degrees. Push heel away. Exhale, lower leg. Increase strength by holding leg at 90, 60, 30 degrees for one breath. Reverse, then do both legs.

5. Because it may be confusing to see how these three leg lifts differ, here is a picture of all three variations. First, both legs bend; then only one leg bends; third, both legs are straight throughout.

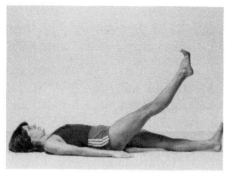
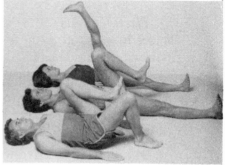

Leg Lifts: Both Legs Straight Throughout   Compare: Three Variations on Leg Lifts

6. Pose. Upward Stretched Out Feet Pose (Urdhva Prasarita Padasana). Exhale, press lower back to floor and lift both legs to 90 degrees. Exhale, lower legs to 60 degrees, hold for one breath. Exhale, lower legs to 30 degrees, hold for one breath. Exhale, lower legs. When strength has increased, lift legs to 30, 60, 90 degrees with holds. Slowly increase holds. Eventually do pose with arms stretched overhead on floor.

Benefits: Strengthens stomach and back.

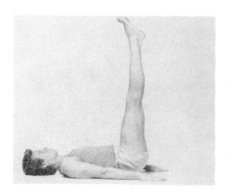
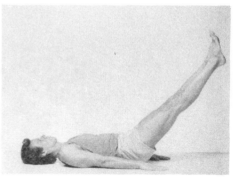
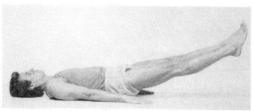

Clockwise From Top Left: Upward Stretched Out Feet-90°; 60°; 30°

SIT-UPS

1. Placement. Lie on your back. Bend your knees, place feet parallel to each other on a wall. Cross your arms and hold each elbow with opposite hand.

2. Variation. Exhale, tuck the chin to the chest and lift the head and the upper back, one vertebra at a time off the floor. Shoulders are low, away from ears. Lift with control, lower with control. As with stretching, never jerk.

3. Variation. Begin as in No. 1. Interlace fingers behind head. Exhale, roll head and upper back up as in No. 2. Flex hips and touch the elbows to thighs above the knees. Place toes on wall, lower the upper back, but do not place head to floor. Contract the stomach again, repeating exercise. Begin by doing 2 or 3, work up to 10.

4. Variation. To strengthen the oblique muscles begin as in No. 3 with toes on wall. Flex as in No. 3, but cross the right elbow to touch the left knee, then cross the left elbow to right knee. Release by placing toes on wall, upper back down, head lifted. Repeat as many times as possible without strain, remembering that it's the elbows that cross, not the knees.

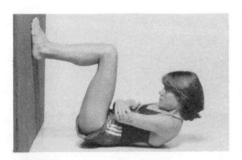
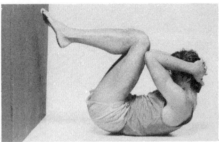
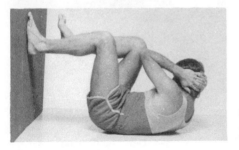

Clockwise From Top Left: Sit-Ups-Hands Across Chest; Elbows to Knees; Sit-Ups-Elbow to Opposite Knee

Benefits: Strengthens neck and stomach, protects back. People with swaybacks should do these regularly.

BOAT POSE

(Navasana)

1. Placement. Sit in the Stick Pose (see p. 169). Draw your knees up to your chest, exhale, lift feet slightly off the floor, wrapping arms around shins. Balance on sitting bones, back erect.

2. Pose. Exhale, push heels up and away, keeping legs straight with feet and knees together. Keep breathing. Extend arms along body parallel to floor, palms in. Open chest by keeping shoulders away from ears, lifting sternum (breastbone) to ceiling. *Balance forward on sitting bones and not back on the sacrum or lower back.* Release to Stick Pose after holding for a few breaths.

3. Variation. Do No. 1. Exhale, push heels away, extending legs as in No. 2, but support backs of knees with hands. Use arms as levers to help open the chest and keep back concave by doing gentle dog tilt with pelvis. *Do not fall backwards on lower back.*

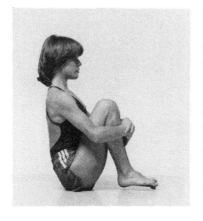
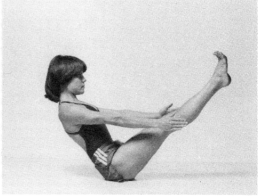

Boat Pose-Placement   Boat Pose

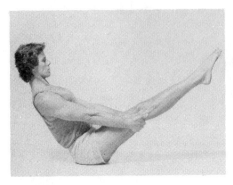

Boat Pose-Hands Supporting Legs

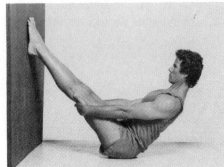

Boat Pose Against Wall

4. Aid. Sit on a mat facing a wall. Place feet on the wall so the heels are level with the eyes. Place hands behind the knees and lean back until the torso is at a right angle to the legs. When balance increases, let go of legs, turn palms in.

Caution: *Do not attempt this pose if you have a weak lower back.*

Benefits: Strengthens back and abdominal area, opens chest, stretches legs.

9

Don't Be Girdled: Poses for Shoulders and Arms

Runners sometimes concentrate so much on their lower body that the chest, shoulders and arms remain underdeveloped unless specific work is done on this area. A weak upper body taxes the lower body by making it work harder to carry and balance a dull torso. Such imbalanced development can lead to a stiff shoulder girdle with a concave chest, a tension-prone neck, and weak, unresponsive arms. In addition, "cement" shoulders—those stiff and immovable joints—can cause discomfort and painful injury.

Focusing on the shoulders and arms in your yoga practice can therefore be very helpful. This section includes exercises and postures to benefit the upper back, shoulders, and arms. A special caution should be noted for two of these exercises, push-ups and pull-ups. These exercises benefit athletes by developing the arms and strengthening the abdomen. However, some athletes should do only a moderate number of push-ups, and increase their time doing work to stretch the stomach. Tight stomachs act as levers on the chest, pulling the rib cage down. The chest becomes flat and lifeless, and the breath is limited. Usually the head will protrude also. When the chest is collapsed, the back muscles lose tone because they are always extended. The whole body loses balance. Look in the mirror. If you tend toward this pattern, alter your exercises to make yourself truly balanced and fit, not just hard. (Do fewer push-ups, leg lifts, and sit-ups. Do more back-bending poses.)

As you do the following exercises observe the face, throat, and arms and allow these areas to remain soft and passive. Remember that as the shoulders, arms and the thoraxic spine become stronger and more flexible, the chest can open. Deeper, freer breathing will result. Liberating your breath means longer, stronger runs and more challenging workouts.

CHEST OPENER

1. Placement. Stand square to a wall. Feet are parallel and apart under hips. With wrists at eye-level, place hands on wall, shoulder width apart, mid-finger vertical. Walk back until your arms are fully extended and legs perpendicular to floor.

2. Pose. Exhale. *Keeping arms straight, and without moving hands,* turn inner elbow down and under. Do *dog-tilt.* Sternum moves toward wall, eyes look straight ahead. Legs remain perpendicular with *kneecaps up* and *arms straight*. Hold for several breaths, release by walking into wall.

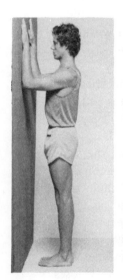
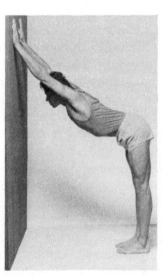
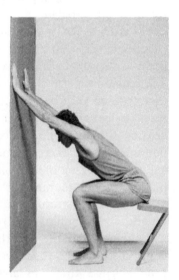

Chest Opener
-Placement

Chest Opener

Seated in Chair

3. Variation. The higher the hands are placed on the wall, the more the shoulders are worked. Therefore begin with the hands placed at shoulder level if position in No. 1 causes the arms to bend. Gradually work hands back up as the shoulders become looser.

4. Aid. If tight legs prevent you from doing the above with straight legs, sit in a chair facing wall. Do No. 2.

Benefits: Loosens shoulders, stretches legs. Strengthens arms, upper back and chest.

HAND CLASP SHOULDER STRETCH

1. Placement. Stand in Mountain Pose. Interlace fingers behind your back.

2. Pose. Move both hands to the left, placing back of right hand against left rib cage. Exhale, lower the shoulders, and draw shoulder blades together and down. The left elbow moves in toward the spine and down. Breathe high into the chest and lift the spine with each inhalation. Hold 15 to 20 seconds. Reverse.

Benefits: Stretches chest, strengthens upper back, adds mobility to shoulder girdle.

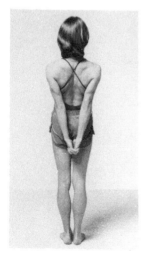 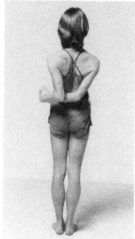

From Left: Hand Clasp Shoulder Stretch-Placement; Hand Clasp Shoulder Stretch

ARM STRETCH

(Parvatasana)

1. Placement. Sit in Hero's Pose (see p. 87), or, if this is too difficult at first, stand with your feet parallel and one foot apart. Interlock your fingers with the right thumb on top.

2. Pose. Exhale, extend your arms straight up, pushing the palms to the ceiling, *maintaining the interlock.* Soften the face, throat as you continue elongating both sides evenly. Hold for 10 seconds, release, change the interlock by shifting the fingers so that the left thumb is on top; repeat.

3. Variation. If you are standing, note that although the feet are apart, the body remains in Mountain Pose. Stretch the arms, but keep the face and throat passive.

4. Aid. In position 1, hold a tie between your hands, keeping the hands shoulder width apart. Exhale, stretching the arms upward alongside the ears, pushing your fists to the ceiling. Keep the tension on the tie by walking your hands in slightly to the center if necessary.

Benefits: Strengthens and loosens shoulders and upper arms. Particularly good stretch for hands and knees.

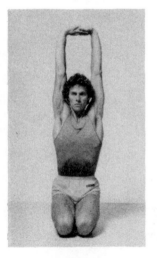
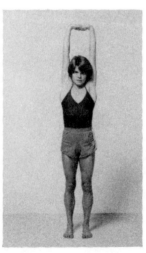
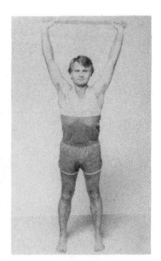

Arm Stretch-Pose   Standing-Arm Stretch   Arm Stretch with Tie

WRIST STRETCH

1. Placement. Stand facing a wall. Bend the arms at the elbows, turn the palms down so fingers point to floor. Place fingers and as much of palm as possible on the wall.

2. Pose. On each exhalation lean more heavily into the hands, trying to get the entire palm on the wall. As flexibility increases, move hands higher up the wall.

Benefits: Increases flexibility in wrists.

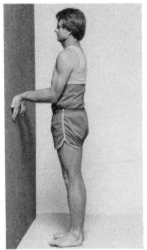
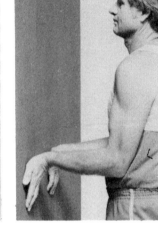

Wrist Stretch-Placement   Wrist Stretch

COW'S FACE-ARMS ONLY

(Gomukasana)

1. Placement. Sit in Hero's Pose (see p. 87). Distribute the weight evenly on both buttocks.

2. Pose. Exhale, bend the left arm and place the left hand on the spine, palm out. Keep left shoulder down and back. Stretch the fingers up. Exhale, extend the right arm straight up along the

ear. Maintain the right arm's stretch as you bend it at the elbow
and grasp the left hand with the right. Keep the spine straight,
shoulders level and back. Hold for 10 to 15 seconds, reverse.

3. Variation. Do not be concerned with touching the hands. The
important point is to minimize the disturbance of your Hero's
Pose, so check your feet, hips, shoulders, throat, and face as you
bend the arms.

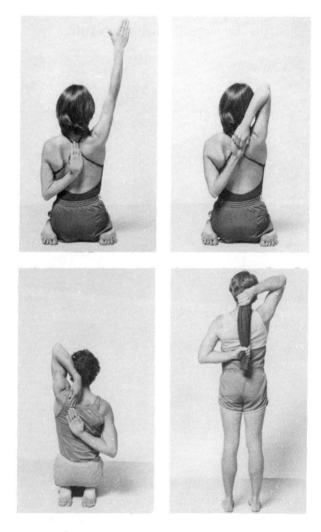

Left to Right From Top: Cow's Face-Arms Only-Preparation;
Cow's Face-Arms Only; Modified Pose; Cow's Face with Towel

4. Aid. You may practice this pose standing. Hold a towel, rope or belt in your right hand and reach for it with the left. Use the towel as a link between the two hands.

Benefits: Excellent for people with rounded shoulders, concave chests, tight arms.

PUSH-UPS

1. Placement. Lie face down on floor, feet a foot apart. Place hands under shoulders, fingers spread, middle fingers parallel. Keep the elbows close to the body, arms parallel to each other throughout. Bend knees and bring heels toward buttocks.

2. Pose. Lift torso off floor, do a cat tilt. Keep the back as a unit throughout. Inhale, press evenly on the inside and outside of the palms and straighten the arms. Exhale, bend elbows and lower the body. Touch only the chest to the floor. Repeat. Never at any time allow the back to arch. Do as many as you can without strain. Build to 10.

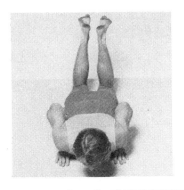
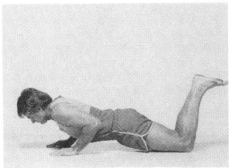
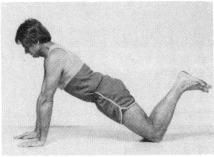

Clockwise from Top Left: Push-Ups-Bent Knee-Placement; Torso Lifted for Push-Ups; Completed Push-Ups

3. Variation. If you can't do one push-up begin on hands and knees, bring heels to buttocks. Come into the push-up position. Exhale, bend the elbows and lower the body. Roll to one side, pull knees to chest, use hands to lift yourself to bent-knee push-up position. By doing "push-downs" you will gain strength to do push-ups.

4. Variation. When you have sufficient strength, do full body push-ups. By keeping the elbows close to the body you will build balanced strength in the arms. Keep the pelvis tucked in cat tilt, kneecaps pulled up. For greater difficulty move the palms toward the feet.

Benefits: Builds strength in arms and stomach and increases mobility in wrists.

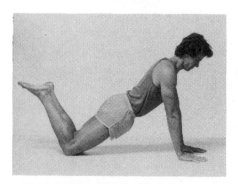
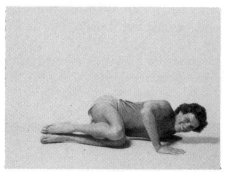
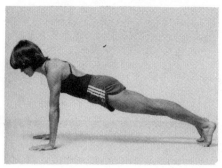

Clockwise from Top Left: Begin Here for Weak Arms; Getting Up; Full Body Push-Up

CHAIR PUSH-UPS

1. Placement. Place the back of a chair against a wall. Kneel arm's length away and place heel of hands on seat of chair, fingers parallel to each other. Bend elbows and lower chest to chair. Straighten legs so you are on toes and hands. Pelvis is tucked in cat tilt.

2. Pose. With your elbows in next to the body, exhale, and straighten the arms. Shoulders are low, away from ears throughout. Keep head in line with body, touch chest to chair, not nose. Inhale down. Do as many as you can with this alignment.

Benefits: Strengthens arms, wrists, shoulders, abdomen.

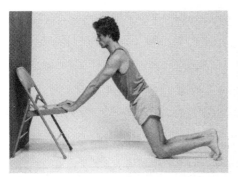
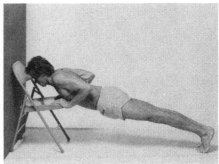
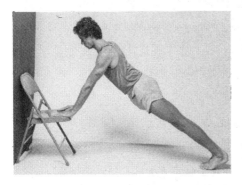

Clockwise from Top Left: Chair Push-Ups-Placement; Placement with Straight Legs; Chair Push-Up

TABLE PULL-UPS

1. Placement. Sit under a sturdy table, buttocks in line with table edge. Lean back slightly and hold table with both hands, shoulder width apart, palms in.

2. Pose. Lift torso to plank position, tuck pelvis in cat tilt so you are suspended by hands and supported on heels. Exhale, bend the elbows and pull up until head touches table. Work to 10 or more.

3. Variation. Sit under table with legs under the table, buttocks in line with table edge. Lean back and hold table edge with both hands, back of palms facing you. Proceed as in No. 2. This works different arm muscles than No. 2.

Benefits: Strengthens wrists, elbows, arms, shoulders, stomach. Prepares for hanging pull-ups.

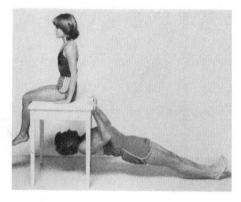

Table Pull-Up-Pose

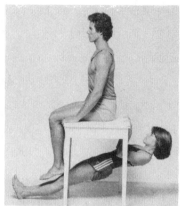

Reversed Hand Hold

INTENSE FRONT STRETCH

(Purvottanasana)

1. Placement. Sit in Stick Pose (see p. 169). Bend the knees enough to place the feet flat on the floor, slightly apart. (Eventually keep feet together.) Knees directly in line with feet, not dropped out to sides. Keep feet parallel.

2. Pose. Exhale, straighten the arms and legs and lift the body toward the ceiling. Buttocks contracted and in cat tilt. Press the soles of the feet flat to the floor but do not allow the toes to angle in. Stretch the chest open and let the head drop back. Hold for a few breaths, gradually increase time. Release back to Stick Pose.

3. Variation. Do No. 2, but instead of balancing on the soles of the feet, work on the heels for a few seconds. Then exhale and stretch the soles to the floor.

4. Aid. If the arms and shoulders are too weak to balance, use a bench under the buttocks to support some of the weight.

5. Aid. Occasionally work with the toes pushing against a wall to help keep the legs straight. Press solidly on the joint under the big toe; it will stretch the inner ankle.

Caution: *Do not do this pose if you have a neck problem.*

Benefits: Stretches feet, ankles, chest. Strengthens buttocks, feet, legs, shoulders and arms.

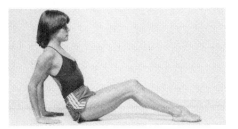 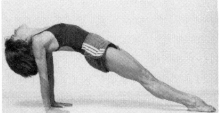

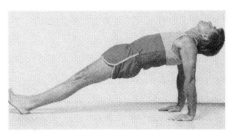 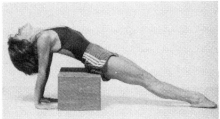

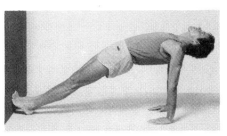

Left to Right from Top: Intense Front Stretch-Placement; Intense Front Stretch; On Heels; Supported Front Stretch; Toes Against Wall

10

Foundation: Poses for the Feet, Knees, and Lower Legs

Between the fashion industry and Cinderella our feet have been terribly abused. All too frequently we sacrifice foot comfort for styles of tortuous extremes: high heels, pointed toes, hard unyielding surfaces. And the wondrous tale of Cinderella has etched into our minds that somehow small feet are irretrievably linked with beauty, benevolence, kingliness. Large feet are reserved for the awkward "uglies" who will always be denied true refinement and grace. We have been sold a horrible, unhealthy bill of goods.

The twenty-six bones of the feet need adequate space to distribute and balance the weight of the body. Lack of space leads to certain bones, muscles, tendons, ligaments being over-used or under-used. The whole body must shift to accommodate its base.

Encourage your feet to expand to their normal size and shape. See to it that both socks and shoes allow space for the toes to spread. Every now and then cajole or pay someone to massage your feet. The kind person will be repaid by your "foot-felt" eternal gratitude. Another way to bring health to the feet is by stretching them.

When the feet are exercised the legs, knees and hips must be involved. The arches of the feet are lifted by the muscles of the lower legs. Imbalance in these muscles can affect not only the arches of the feet but influence the position of the ankle. An aberration here necessitates a compensation by either the knees, or the hips, or both.

Most problems of the feet are mechanical. Proper movement (exercise) may be the fastest, most effective route to remedies. Try all of these poses and work often but gently on the ones that reveal your greatest tightnesses. Practicing the many variations of the Hero's Pose will probably bring the most benefits. This pose brings balance to the feet and ankles, stretches the knees, and revitalizes the legs. Along with the Shoulder Stand, the Hero's Pose is highly recommended for relief of fatigue in the legs.

FINGERS AND TOES ENTWINED

1. Placement. Sit on the floor or in chair. Bend the right knee out, hold the right foot with both hands. Interlace the fingers of the left hand with the toes of the right foot. Place the base of the fingers into the base of the toes.

2. Pose. To increase the stretch, push the heel out, press with the left hand and stretch the toes toward the right knee. Hold 15 to 20 seconds; reverse.

3. Variation. If you can't get the fingers between the toes, place the heel of the right hand on the balls of the foot and wrap the fingers over the top of the toes. Extend the heel and by pressing with the right hand curl the toes toward the knee. Hold, then repeat with right foot and left hand.

Benefits: Spreads toes and bones of feet.

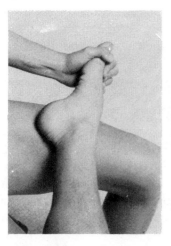
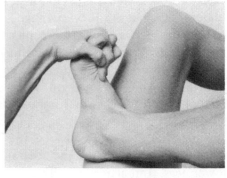

From Left: Fingers and Toes Entwined-Placement; Stretching Toes, Sole, Heel

FOOT EXTENSION

1. Placement.   Lie on back. Bend left knee, place left foot on floor. Bend right knee into chest. Then extend right leg until it is almost straight; press heel toward ceiling. Relax face, neck, arms.

2. Pose. Push heel out, then ball of foot, then toes. Reverse action by curling toes back toward knee and extending ball of foot. Once again push heel out. Roll foot from position to position repeating full cycle three times. Do same action with leg at 60 degrees and 30 degrees. Reverse legs. Then do entire cycle with the working leg straight as foot stretches.

Benefits: Strengthens arches, stretches feet and ankles, brings awareness to feet.

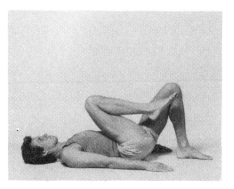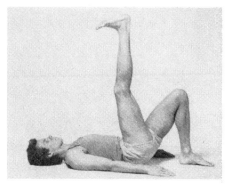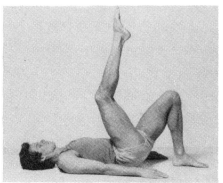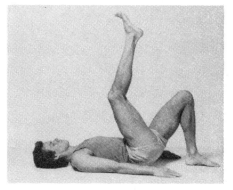

Clockwise from Top Left: Foot Extension-Preparation for Placement; Placement with Heel Extended; Pose with Ball of Foot Extended; Pose with Toes Pointed

FOOT CIRCLES

1. Placement. Lie on back. With left leg bent, put left foot on floor below buttock. Lift right leg toward ceiling; the leg may be slightly bent. Relax face and neck.

2. Pose. Curl toes of right foot back toward knee. Spread toes apart, push heel toward ceiling. Circle toes and entire foot to far right, then point toes toward ceiling; then circle toes to left. Continue three circles to right, then reverse circles going to the left first. Change feet and repeat entire cycle.

Benefits: Brings mobility to ankles, stretches feet, strengthens stomach and back.

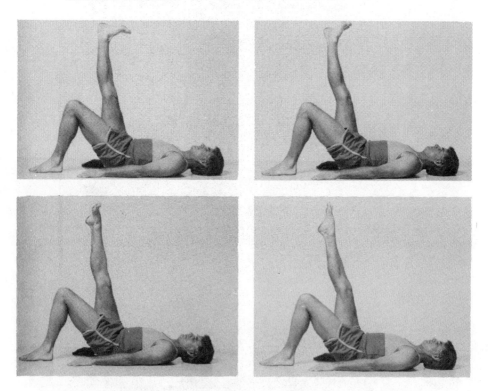

Clockwise from Top Left: Foot Circles-Placement; Foot Rotates to Right; Toes Pointed; Foot Rotates to Left

The next four poses make up a series of stretches that are excellent for the feet and legs. These poses are known as the Squat

Series. Study and practice them individually first. The following photos show the complete sequence as it should be done. After completing the sequence, reverse the series. Repeat the series four times to warm up. Once your muscles are warmed up hold each pose 10 to 30 seconds.

PREPARATION FOR HERO'S POSE–SQUAT SERIES POSE I

(Virasana)

1. Placement. On hands and knees place inner edges of legs and feet together. Toes are pointed so front of feet and ankles are on the floor.

2. Pose. Exhale and *slowly* walk your hands toward your knees as you sit back on your heels. Stretch back the inner edges of the feet, keeping contact between them. Sit upright making the back long. Place hands on thighs. Hold 15 to 20 seconds. Build to two minutes.

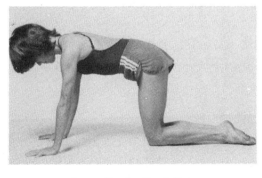

Preparation for Hero's Pose

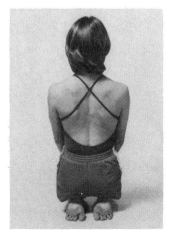

Hero's Pose (Squat Series Pose I)

3. Variation. Most people can't do this pose with the heels together. If your heels come apart, go back to placement No. 1, separate the feet but keep them straight. Do not allow the heels to angle out or toes to point in. Keep this alignment and again sit on heels. Let weight of body stretch front of feet and ankles.

4. Aid. If the front of your ankles don't touch the floor, place a rolled towel or small cushion under them. The cushion should be low enough to allow stretching but high enough for support. You should be *almost* comfortable. If necessary combine this with the following aid.

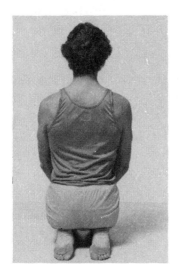

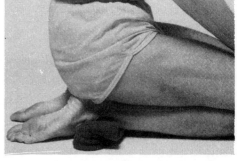

Ankles supported in preparation for Hero's Pose

Feet separated but parallel

5. Aid. If your knees are very tight and the buttocks will not meet the heels, place a rolled towel or cushion above the heels and under the buttocks. This is important to protect the knees from stretching too fast. Again, the cushion should be of the size that makes you almost comfortable.

6. Aid. If one or both of your knees hurt take the corner of a washcloth or a rope and place it behind the knee. As you sit back into the pose hold the rope tight into the joint. This makes more space in the joint and frequently will make the difference between effective and painful stretching. *Never hold a pose with pain in the knees.*

7. *Variation.* An excellent series for stretching and warming up the feet is the Preparation for Hero's Pose, followed by the next three poses. Then reverse the series. Repeat four times, then hold each pose as prescribed.

Benefits: Brings balance to the feet and ankles. Stretches feet, ankles, lower leg, and knees.

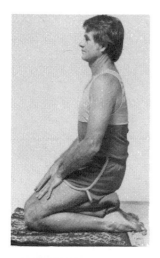
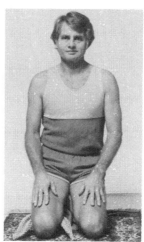
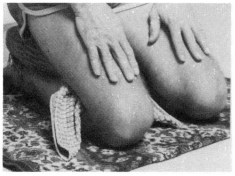

Clockwise from Top Left: Buttocks supported in Preparation for Hero's Pose; Support in Knee Joint-Preparation for Hero's Pose; Close-Up of Towel in Knee Joint

KNEELING FOOT STRETCH—SQUAT SERIES POSE II

1. Placement. Begin in Preparation for Hero's Pose (see p. 81). Turn toes under. Use your hands to help turn the toes so all ten are on floor. Heels are directly above toes.

2. Pose. Sit on heels, torso upright. Be sure lower back is long with gentle curve into the body. Now, let the weight of the body settle into the feet. Hold just a breath or two, build to 1 to 2 minutes.

Benefits: Stretches soles of feet.

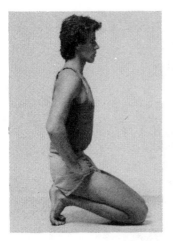

Kneeling Foot Stretch-Placement

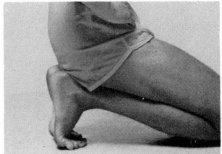

Close-up of Feet

BENT KNEE FOOT BALANCE—SQUAT SERIES POSE III

1. Placement. Begin in Kneeling Foot Stretch, except raise arms to horizontal position straight in front of shoulders.

2. Pose. Exhale, lift knees from floor, thighs parallel to floor. Buttocks remain on heels. Hold and breathe. Continue to next pose.

Benefits: Brings mobility to feet and knees. Balancing poses give poise.

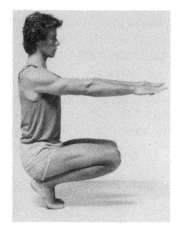

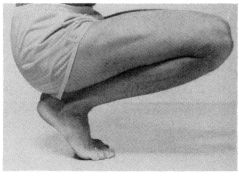

Left to Right: Bent Knee Foot Balance-Pose; Close-up of Feet

SQUAT—SQUAT SERIES POSE IV

1. Placement. Begin in Bent Knee Foot Balance.

2. Pose. Exhale, stretch heels back to floor. Bring knees as far forward as possible to stretch the Achilles tendon. The back will round slightly to facilitate balance. Hold 15 to 20 seconds. To warm up feet, reverse series. Repeat series four times, then hold each pose as described.

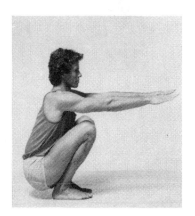

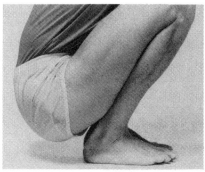

Close-up of Feet

Squat-Pose (Series IV)

3. Variation. Stand with feet under hips, face a partner. Both people extend arms forward from shoulders, grasp each other's wrists. Exhale, bend knees, round back, squat with heels on floor. Hold and breathe. To increase stretch, back away from partner. Knees continue to move toward floor. Stand to release.

4. Variation. Stand arm's length away from a sink, window sill, or the two knobs of an open door. Grasp edge with both hands. Feet parallel under hips. Exhale, bend the knees and squat, keep heels on floor. Work knees toward floor. Tilt pelvis in dog tilt. Hold for one to two minutes.

5. Variation. Stand with back 8 to 12 inches from wall. Bend knees and squat. Bend elbows and press them into wall. Press heels down and lengthen spine, open chest. Use hands to press thighs forward, bringing them to a more horizontal position. Hold 10 to 15 seconds. Slowly increase time.

Benefits: Stretches Achilles tendon, strengthens front of leg, relieves tension in lower back.

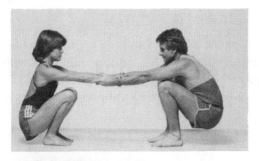

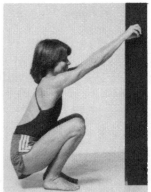

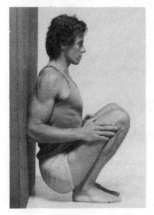

Clockwise from Top Left: Squat with Partner; Squat Using Door; Squat Against Wall

HERO'S POSE
(Virasana)

1. Placement. Kneel, knees together, feet separated enough to set buttocks on floor between feet. Do not allow the toes to angle in toward each other. Keep stretching the inner ankle and foot straight back.

2. Pose. Exhale, lower the buttocks to the floor. Sit up tall, place hands on thighs, close to knees. Breathe normally and hold 15 to 20 seconds. Slowly build time. Release, bring legs forward, if necessary massage knees with hands then straighten legs to tighten kneecaps.

3. Variation. Begin as in No. 1. Take hold of calf muscles and roll the muscles away from the midline of the body. Hold muscles this way as you sit in No. 2. This removes the bulk of the muscle out of the way and allows the knee joint to close further.

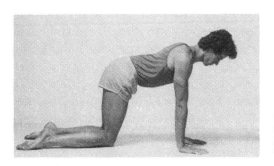

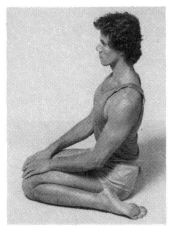

Left to Right From Top: Hero's Pose-Placement; Hero's Pose-Side View; Hero's Pose Viewed from Back

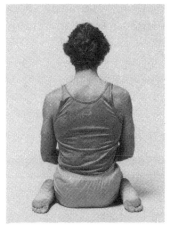

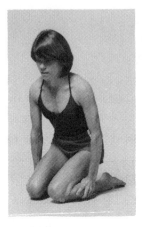 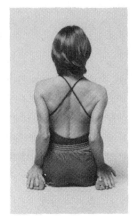

Entering Hero's Pose by   Palms on Feet
Rolling Calves Out

4. Variation. Once in the pose, turn the hands away from the midline of the body so fingers point directly back. Place the palms on the soles of each foot. Press the little toe side of the foot and flatten the entire front of the foot into the floor. Hold and breathe. This helps to straighten the kneecaps which should be vertical.

5. Aid. If the knees are too uncomfortable in this pose sit on a rolled towel, mat or cushion. The amount of lift under the buttocks should be determined by how you feel. You should feel stretch in the knees, but not pain.

6. Aid. As in Preparation for Hero's Pose (see p. 81) use a rope or washcloth behind the knee joint to relieve pressure in knees. You also may need to raise the buttocks as in No. 4 above.

Benefits: The best pose to bring balance to feet. Excellent for relieving fatigue in legs.

RECLINING HERO
(Supta Virasana)

1. Placement. Sit in Hero's Pose (see p. 87). If sitting on the floor between the feet is possible, proceed to this pose.

2. Pose. Exhale, lean back and support yourself on the hands, then on both elbows and forearms. *Tuck the pelvis in cat tilt.* Drop the head back so top of head rests on floor. Then bring the chin toward the chest until face is parallel to floor. Extend the arms straight along the ears, palms up, knees together. On exhalations stretch the arms as you move the lower back toward the floor. Continue for several breaths, gradually increasing your time. Come up using the elbows again.

3. Variation. In the beginning, simply lower your back and extend the arms, hold for a few seconds and come up carefully. Allow the knees to separate in the pose. Do not attempt to flatten the lower back; see instead if it will soften on its own.

4. Aid. If this pose is impossible, use pillows or blankets to support the back. The pillows should be positioned just below the waist and extend to support the head. Modify the height of the support according to your degree of flexibility. You should be *almost* comfortable.

Benefits: Stretches and aligns feet, lower legs and thighs. Stretches spine.

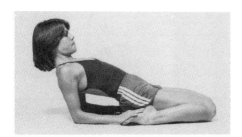
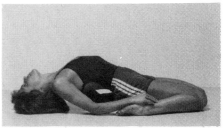
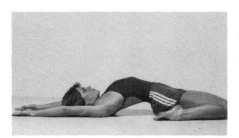
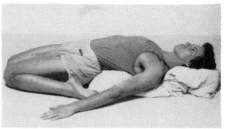

Left to Right From Top: Reclining Hero-Entering Pose on Forearms; Head Drops Back; Full Reclining Hero-Arms Overhead; Supported Reclining Hero

SINK STRETCH FOR ACHILLES AND CALVES

1. Placement. Stand in Mountain Pose, arm's length from and holding a sink, open car window, fence, or two knobs of open door. Tuck pelvis down in cat tilt.

2. Pose. Exhale, bend elbows and lean into sink. Keep body straight from head to heels, which remain on floor. Repeat 10 times; last time hold 10 to 15 seconds.

3. To intensify, continue to hold ledge and with knees tight and back straight, exhale and bend at the hips. Stretch the buttocks away from your hands. Relax neck by letting head hang. Inhale, stand. Repeat No. 2 then No. 3 several times. Finish in No. 3 then lift feet off floor so you are on your heels.

Benefits: Stretches Achilles tendon, calves, and back.

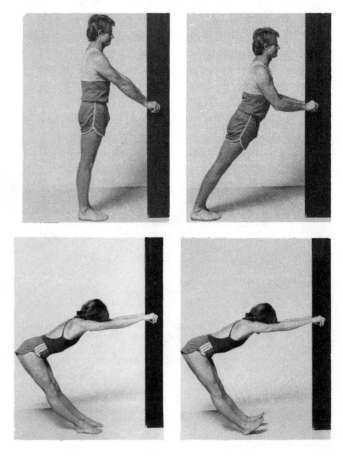

Left to Right
From Top:
Sink Stretch
Placement; Pose;
Bending at Hips;
on Heels

ACHILLES, CALF STRETCH

1. Placement. Face a wall. Turn the right foot so the toes rest on the wall and the heel is on the floor. Step back 3 feet with the left foot, toes pointing directly forward. Place hands on wall opposite shoulders, arms straight. Lift left heel and square hips to wall.

2. Pose. Hold the above and step solidly on left heel with both kneecaps tight. Tuck pelvis down firmly in cat tilt. The entire body should be square to the wall so there is equal pressure on both hands. Hold 10 to 15 seconds. Reverse.

3. Variation. To increase stretch, bend the right knee toward wall. Keep left knee tight, tail tucked firmly, open chest. If lower back hurts move entire torso forward by bending elbows, tuck pelvis in cat tilt more firmly.

Benefits: Marvelous stretch for lower legs, ankles, calves.

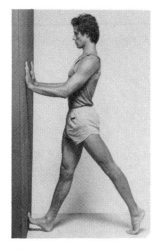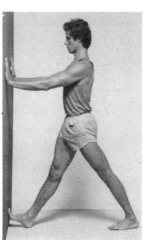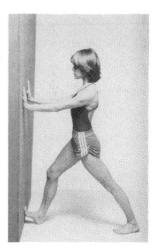

Achilles, Calf Stretch-Placement   Pose   Variation-Knee Bent

11

The Key to Posture:
Hips and Thighs

The hip socket is formed where the pelvis and the thigh bone (femur) meet. This is the joint by which the leg is tied to the body; its complexity is indicated in the accompanying diagrams.

Note that the muscles which support and move the hip socket are connected to several places: the front of the spine, the hip bones, the sitting bones, the lower back, the thigh bones, and below the knees at the lower leg. Underlying these muscles are more muscles and numerous ligaments that further stabilize the hip joint. (See p. 94-95.)

As stated earlier, the tilt of the pelvis determines the curves of the back. In turn, the tilt of the pelvis is determined by how the thigh bone and pelvis fit together. If the muscles, ligaments or tendons that join the leg to the body are too loose or too tight, they will affect how the pelvis rests on the thigh bones.

If the connective tissue around the hip socket is strong and flexible, the pelvic bones (where you put your hands on your hips) will be horizontal and symmetrical. Such balance in the pelvis insures adequate space for the entire contents of the pelvic bowl, the viscera; it also decreases the chances of illness resulting from the stagnation of body fluids or the compression of nerves and organs.

In this chapter there are poses for the front of the hip (the groin area) and for the adductors, which are muscles that draw the

93

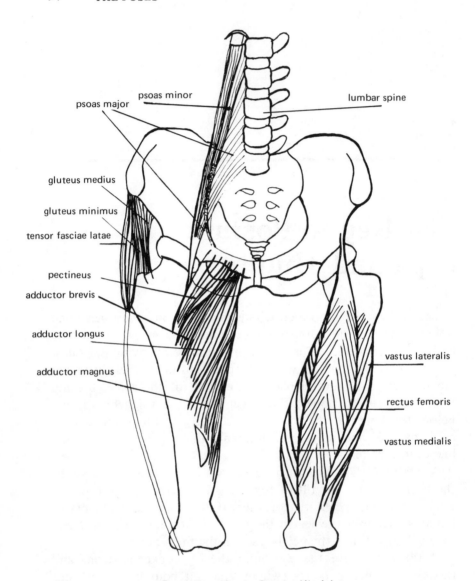

psoas minor

psoas major

lumbar spine

gluteus medius

gluteus minimus

tensor fasciae latae

pectineus

adductor brevis

adductor longus

adductor magnus

vastus lateralis

rectus femoris

vastus medialis

Front View: Muscles Crossing Hip Joint

legs together. The Gate Pose (Parighasana) stretches the sides of
the hips. Due to the variety of muscles around the hip socket,
many stretches for other muscles of this area are contained in
other chapters.

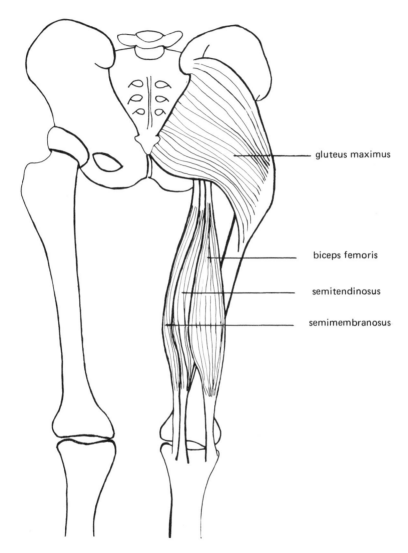

Back View Buttock Muscles and Hamstrings Crossing Hip Socket

A simple way to increase flexibility in the hips is to sit on the floor more often! (If you are very tight the floor will be uncomfortable at first so get a big cushion. Sit on this regularly and in no time you'll be comfortable on the floor.) The hip is capable of an enormous range of movement, none of which is encouraged by modern chairs. Just sitting with crossed legs rotates the hip socket, stretches the inner thighs, and flexes the knees. So get out of the soft chair!

Two cautions: The muscle that crosses the front of the hip, the quadriceps femoris, also crosses the knee. So does the fascia lata. Move into and out of the poses slowly to give yourself a chance to prevent any undue stretch in the knee. It's such an unforgiving joint. Also, to stretch the groin area, many times the torso must lean backward into an arch. To protect the lower back always *tuck the pelvis in the cat tilt and lengthen the entire spine.* (See Chapter 15 on backbending.)

TAILOR POSE

1. Placement. Sit in Stick Pose (see p. 169). Bend both legs and cross the ankles.

2. Pose. Exhale, bring the ankles in toward the groins. Use the hands to move the feet under the thighs so that the soles of the feet are in line with the outer thighs. Hands rest on knees. Balance evenly on the sitting bones (not on the lower back) as you lift the spine on inhalations. Dog tilt pelvis so spine has four gentle curves. Chin parallel to floor. Release to the Stick Pose after holding 15 to 20 seconds, reverse the legs and repeat.

3. Variation. Do No. 2, stretch the arms straight to ceiling, interlock the fingers. Exhale, press palms to ceiling. Hold for several breaths, release and change interlock position; repeat.

4. Aid. Sit on a pillow in No. 2 to facilitate crossing the legs properly. Using a pillow will help tilt the pelvis slightly forward in dog tilt. The bones at the back of the waist should be slightly indented.

Benefits: Stretches hips, and makes the floor an alternative to chairs!

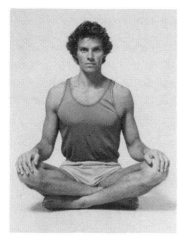

Tailor Pose

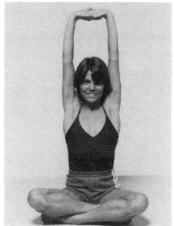

Variation-Palms to Ceiling

BOUND ANGLE

(Badha Konasana)

1. Placement. Sit on floor, bend knees outward and place soles of feet together. Draw feet as close to body as possible. Wrap hands around toes, one hand atop the other. Little toes remain on floor throughout. The spine is long!

2. Pose. Pelvis in dog tilt. This pose works with the breath. On each inhalation the entire spine lifts, grows. With each exhalation the legs soften toward the ground. This is a pose for the hips, not the knees; relax in the groin area. Hold 15 seconds, build to 2 minutes, then hold as long as you can.

3. Aid. Have a partner sit opposite you on the floor. Once in the pose the partner rests his or her legs on your thighs. The partner does not push, just rests. Breathe to lengthen the spine, breathe to soften the groins.

4. Aid. If the back bones at the waist poke out, you need to raise the buttocks. Sit on a cushion or rolled towel. You may also sit with your back against a wall with or without the cushion.

Without over-arching the back, lengthen the front of the body and the spine by doing the dog tilt with the pelvis.

5. Aid. Learn to do this pose with the back extended by using a wall. Lie in Stick Pose, legs stretching up a wall (see p. 169). Bend the knees outward, bring the soles of the feet together; with your hands on the lower legs pull the feet as close to the body as possible. Gently press the thighs back toward the wall.

Benefits: Excellent for health of pelvic region. Stretches inner legs, increases mobility of hips.

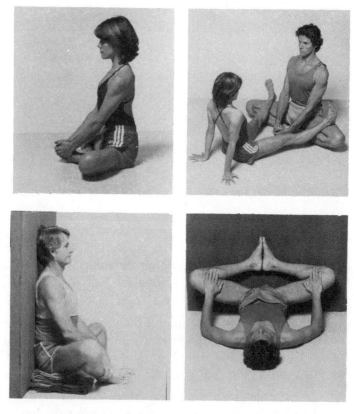

Left to Right From Top: Bound Angle-Pose; Weight on Legs; Against Wall with Buttocks Raised; On Back Against Wall

PREPARATION FOR HALF LOTUS

1. Placement. Sit in Stick Pose (see p. 169). Bend right knee up so heel is close to body. Let knee drop to side as sole of right foot presses into left thigh. Look at the right foot and see that it is perpendicular to the right lower leg. Keep the foot in this position throughout.

2. Preparation. Put your two hands together, palms up, little fingers together. Using your hands as a scoop pick up the right ankle. Exhale, move the leg to the left, across the body. Do not change the position of the right foot; it should be squared.

3. Pose. Position the foot so the heel is opposite the navel. Pull the heel as close as possible to the navel, then slide the heel into the left hip bone, the foot resting on the groin. *Do not touch the right leg; never press it toward the floor.* Place hands on floor, sit tall and let gravity lower leg as it stretches. Hold 5 to 10 seconds. Build to 30 seconds.

Caution: If your knees hurt, discontinue and consult a teacher.

Benefits: Stretches hips, knees, strengthens ankles, back.

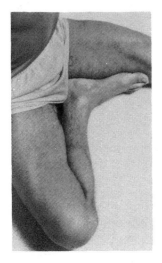

Preparation for Half Lotus-
Foot Placement

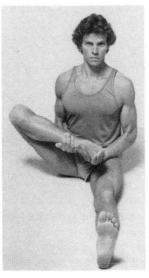

Lower Leg Lifted

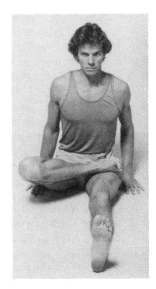

Pose-Foot on Thigh

SINK STRETCH FOR GROIN

1. Placement. Stand 3 feet from ledge. Stand on left foot, place ball of right foot on edge of sink, fence, or desk. Place hands on hips to evaluate if they are level throughout.

2. Pose. Exhale, bend right knee and lean forward. Keep left heel down, tailbone tucked in cat tilt. Repeat 10 times as warm-up, then hold 10 to 15 seconds. Reverse.

Benefits: Versatile groin stretch that can be done frequently.

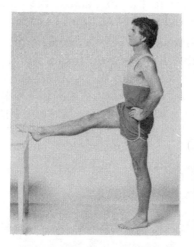
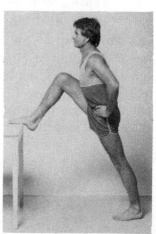

Sink Stretch for Groin-Placement   Pose-Knee Bent

KNEELING GROIN STRETCH

1. Placement. Kneel and bring one leg forward to a 90 degree angle. (When you are more stretched the foot may be further in front of knee.) Interlace fingers and place palms on the forward knee for stability. *Pelvis is in cat tilt.*

2. Pose. Keeping the torso erect, exhale and bend forward knee. Do not allow this leg to go to the side; it should be directly over the toe. Stretch the back leg. Keep this knee turned down. Pelvis must be firmly tucked to protect the back. Hold 15 to 20 seconds.

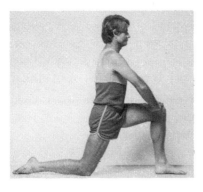
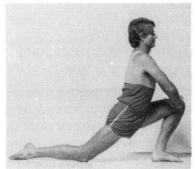

Kneeling Groin Stretch-Placement   Pose

3. Variation. To increase the stretch in the groin, lift both arms overhead, palms in. Tuck pelvis in cat tilt, stretch arms to keep spine long. Slowly bend the forward leg, knee directly over the foot. Achilles tendon is stretched by keeping heel down on forward foot.

4. Variation. To increase the stretch even more, begin in No. 3 and then lift foot of the back leg so the toes point up. If you lose balance do this with one side of your body against a wall. Hold 10 to 15 seconds. *Tuck the tailbone in cat tilt firmly.*

Benefits: Excellent stretch for groin and upper thigh.

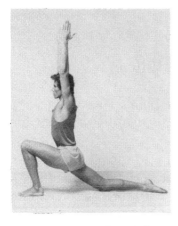
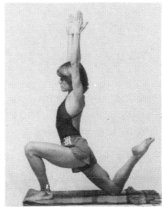

Variation-Arms Extended   Variation-Arms and Lower Leg Lifted

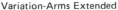

LUNGE GROIN STRETCH

1. Placement. Begin by doing Kneeling Groin Stretch (see p. 100). Stretch torso forward so it rests on forward thigh. Place fingers on floor beside the foot. Turn toes of back foot under.

2. Pose. Tucking pelvis firmly into cat tilt, straighten back knee, pulling kneecap up. Stretch from top of head to back heel. Hold 15 to 20 seconds. Slowly increase time. Reverse.

Benefits: Stretches groin, strengthens legs and back.

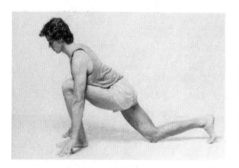 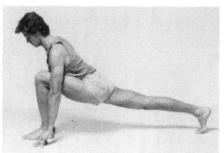

Lunge Groin Stretch-Placement   Pose-Leg Straight

HERO POSE GROIN AND KNEE STRETCH

1. Placement. Sit in Preparation for Hero's Pose (see p. 81). Lean back slightly and place hands on floor so fingers point forward, finger tips in line with toes.

2. Pose. Exhale, tuck the pelvis firmly in cat tilt and lift buttocks from heels. The body is in a slanted plank position. Head is in line with body or dropped back. Hold 10 to 15 seconds. Two cautions: do this very slowly so you don't strain knees. Caution: DO NOT DO POSE IF YOU HAVE AN INJURED NECK.

Benefits: Stretches knees and groin, strengthens back and neck.

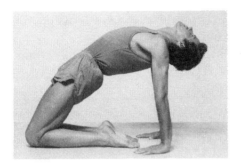

Hero Pose Groin and Knee
Stretch

STANDING HALF BOW

1. Placement. Stand in Mountain Pose, arm's length plus two inches from ledge. Without moving the right foot, balance on right leg and bend left heel to buttock. Hold outside of left ankle with left hand. Stretch right arm forward from shoulder, palm down.

2. Pose. Exhale. Bring torso to horizontal, stretch right arm out on ledge. Lift left leg as high as possible. Keep body level, knee directly back, not out to the side. Hold 15 to 20 seconds. Reverse.

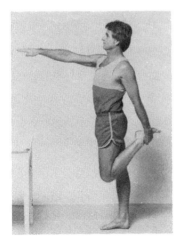

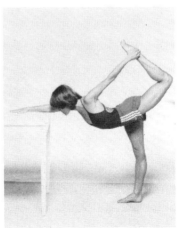

Standing Half Bow-Placement   Pose with Table, Leg Lifting

3. Variation. Do No. 2 above; hold body in horizontal position and bend knee, bringing heel as close to buttock as possible. Be gentle. Hold 15 to 20 seconds. Gradually increase time.

Benefits: Excellent stretch for knees, thighs, and groins. Strengthens back.

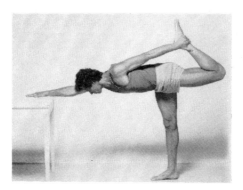

Variation-Heel to Buttock

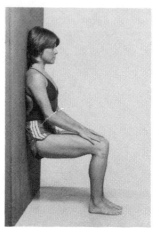

Thigh Strengthener-Pose
(as described below)

THIGH STRENGTHENER

1. Placement. Lean against a wall. Bending at hips, walk your feet out until body is shape of chair. Lower legs are perpendicular to floor so knees are directly above heels, thigh bones are parallel to floor. Tuck pelvis into cat tilt. Relax the belly and neck.

2. Pose. Hold this position. If you have knee problems this pose will probably help but only *if you build time slowly!!!* Begin by holding 10 to 20 seconds for a week. Add five seconds the next week. With this type of caution build to as much as 2 to 4 minutes depending on your needs.

Benefits: Builds strength in thighs, aids knees.

THE GATE

(Parighasana)

1. Placement. Kneel, with inner edges of the legs and feet touching. The feet point back. Place the right heel to the right side, in line with the left knee. Right knee and foot face ceiling. Arms stretch to sides, palms up. Tuck pelvis in cat tilt.

2. Pose. Exhale; with right knee tight, bend sideways at the groin. The back of the right palm will be on the right shin, the left arm stretches overhead. The entire body is lateral. When you have stretched as far as possible, stretch the front of the right foot by pointing the toe. Hold 15 to 20 seconds.

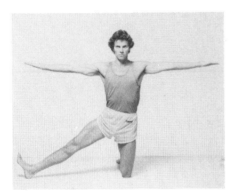
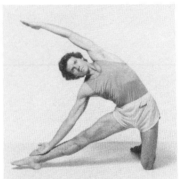
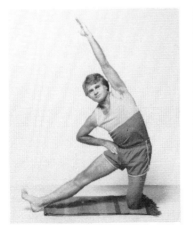
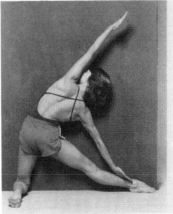

Left to Right From Top: The Gate-Placement; Pose; Hand in Groin; With Wall

3. Variation. Place the right hand, with the thumb away from index finger, into right groin. As you move into the pose press this hand into the body, not down. Feel the hips move to the left as the torso moves to the right.

4. Aid. For correct placement and to help keep the body lateral do this pose with the front of the body against a wall. Shoulders are low even though arms are up.

Benefits: Stretches legs and sides of body, fascial lata particularly.

12

The Screamers:
Hamstring Stretches

The hamstring muscles are aptly named. These muscles contain a high portion of tendon-like fiber; one hamstring, the semi-tendinosus, is fully one-half tendon. Tendons are far less resilient than other muscles, and so are inherently resistant to stretching, like string. This is why the hamstrings require consistent, patient work for athletes who contract these muscles frequently.

The hamstrings cross two joints: the hips and the knees. Therefore the health of the hamstrings influences both of these joints. Proper stretching of the hamstrings can increase the fluidity in the knee, thereby relieving many knee complaints. (See page 95.)

Excess tightness in the hamstrings can affect the back, because these muscles are attached to the sitting bones of the pelvis. If the hamstrings are too tight they literally pull the pelvis down and can cause misalignment in the back, the hips, or the knees. In short, the potentially negative effects of tight hamstrings can't be overemphasized.

Before proceeding to the stretches in this section, do the flexibility test. When lying on your back, raising your leg to a vertical position is considered normal, not average. Even if you are among those who have normal flexibility, do some of these stretches reqularly—hamstrings are always tightening.

Besides stretching the hamstrings before and after every workout, or in a regular yoga practice, try to practice some of these poses throughout the day. The standing poses are most adaptable to this. You can do the Beginner's Hamstring Stretch (see p. 109) easily. When on the phone place one foot on a chair, bend the other knee. Or modify the Scissor Stretch (see p. 113) by simply placing your leg on any support—a desk or table—and hold in that position. Regularity will pay off.

If you have a back problem you particularly need to stretch the hamstrings. The best way for you to stretch your legs is by doing the poses lying on your back. In this way the back is stabilized and the legs must work.

All of these stretches should follow pelvic tilting on hands and knees (see p. 26).

TEST FOR HAMSTRING FLEXIBILITY

1. Placement. Lie on your back in the Mountain Pose.

2. Pose. Keep one leg straight and stretched out; keep the foot squared. Bend the other leg over the chest. Exhale, straighten leg until knee is straight, kneecap up. Keep chin in, neck and arms relaxed; lift the leg as high as possible. The higher the leg, the more flexibility is present. Test other leg. *Perpendicular* legs have normal flexibility.

3. Aid. If you have a bad back do this test by wrapping a towel or belt around the ball of the foot. Hold the ends of the towel with both hands. Have enough length in the towel so your head and shoulders remain on the floor. Straighten both legs, lock the knees.

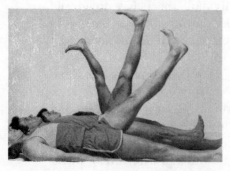

Test for Hamstring Flexibility-Pose

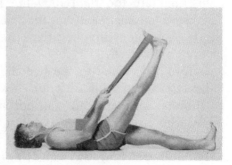

Aid for Bad Backs

Benefits: By stabilizing the back the stretch comes entirely from the hamstrings. This test gives an indication of how often you should stretch hamstrings.

BEGINNER'S HAMSTRING STRETCH

1. Placement. Stand sideways and arm's length away from chair, desk or counter. Place one foot on the seat or back of chair. Straighten this leg and turn knee to face ceiling. Keep hips and shoulders level. Hands on hips. Turn supporting foot out 30 degrees.

2. Pose. Exhale, bend supporting knee directly over toe. By keeping heel down, the Achilles is stretched. Hold 10 to 15 seconds. Exhale, straighten leg. As flexibility increases, raise leg higher.

Benefits: Versatile stretch to do throughout the day. Stretches hamstrings and Achilles tendon.

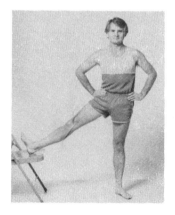

Beginner's Hamstring Stretch-
Placement

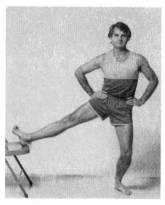

Pose-Supporting Leg Bent

KNEE TO CHEST

1. Placement. Lie on back in Mountain Pose. Bend one knee over chest, interlace fingers and hold leg below knee.

2. Pose. Exhale, squeeze knee into chest. Keep straight leg in original position, do not push off with this heel. Head and shoulders remain on floor. Hold up to 20 seconds. Reverse legs.

3. Variation. Do this pose standing. Begin in Mountain Pose. Bend one knee and lift it high. Bring knee to torso, rather than lowering torso to knee. Interlace fingers under knee and squeeze leg to chest. Keep hip bones level. Hold 20 seconds. Reverse. Stand with back against wall if balance is a problem.

Benefits: Loosens up hamstrings, stretches groin.

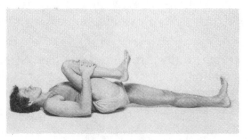
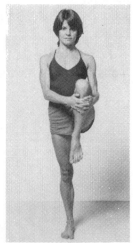

Knee to Chest-Pose; Standing Variation

BEGINNER'S BENT KNEE HAMSTRING STRETCH

1. Placement. Begin on back in Mountain Pose. Bend right leg and place right foot on floor. Bend left knee over the chest. Gently hold behind left knee with both hands.

2. Pose. Exhale, straighten the left leg as far as possible *without lowering the knee.* Extend the heel. Bend leg, then repeat 10 times. Hold last stretch 20 seconds. Reverse.

Benefits: Supports back as hamstrings stretch.

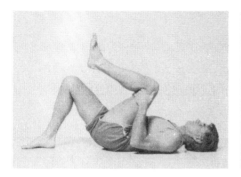
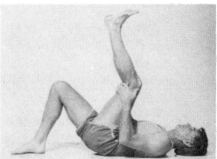

Beginner's Bent Knee Hamstring Stretch-Preparation; Pose

PROGRESSIVE HAMSTRING STRETCH

1. Placement. Lie on back, in Mountain Pose. Toes touch, heels slightly apart, knees straight to ceiling. Bend one leg over chest and wrap towel, sock or shirt around ball of foot.

2. Pose. Exhale, straighten the leg, extend heel. Using the leverage of your arms, bending the elbows out, shoulders on floor, stretch the leg higher and higher. Do not push back of head into floor. Hold at the highest point for 15 to 20 seconds.

Benefits: Excellent way to stretch hamstrings, calves, Achilles tendon while protecting back. When asked which hamstring stretch is most effective, novice stretchers almost always choose this one.

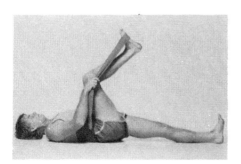
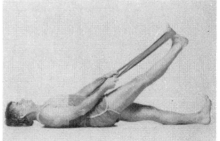

Progressive Hamstring Stretch-Preparation; Pose

SUPINE HAND-TO-FOOT POSE

(Supta Padangusthasana)

1. Placement. Lie on back in Mountain Pose. Bend right knee and grasp big toe with first two fingers and thumb of the right hand. Left hand is on thigh.

2. Pose. Exhale, straighten right knee, heel pushing away from body. The right shoulder remains on the floor. Exhale, bend right elbow out, contract stomach and lift head and upper torso toward leg. Leg stretches further overhead. Place head on knee. Hold two or three breaths. Place head back to ground. Bend right knee, release toe, place foot on floor and straighten leg in Mountain Pose. Reverse.

3. Pose. After doing No. 2 straighten the leg toward ceiling. Exhale, lower leg to the far right. Stretch the inside of the heel. Hold 10 to 15 seconds. Exhale, release. Reverse.

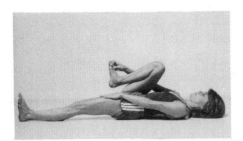 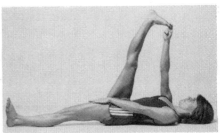

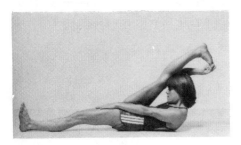 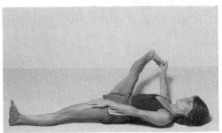

Left To Right From Top: Supine Hand to Foot-Placement; Pose-Leg Straight; Head to Leg; Leg to Side

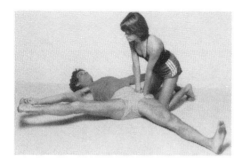

Supine Hand-to-Foot with Partner

4. Aid. Have a partner hold the left hip bone to help you maintain balance in No. 3. Now gravity can be the lever while you give into the stretch. Breathe, hold 15 seconds.

Benefits: Stretches legs, opens hips, strengthens stomach.

SCISSOR STRETCH

1. Placement. Stand in Mountain Pose facing a chair, arm's length away. Lift one leg and place it on the seat or back of a chair depending on your flexibility. Push heel out. Hips are level. Stretch the arms overhead slightly behind the ears, palms in.

2. Pose. Keep the back straight and on exhalation close the torso to the leg like scissors closing. Lift buttocks in dog tilt. At first you won't close very far. Hold at your maximum stretch for 15 seconds. Reverse.

3. Pose. Very few people can do this pose but it is included to show how to do it correctly. It is seen so often with a bent back and collapsed chest.

Benefits: Stretches hamstrings, strengthens back.

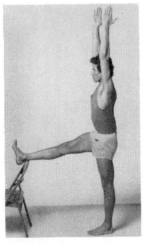
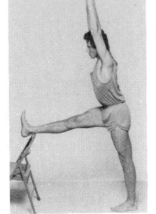
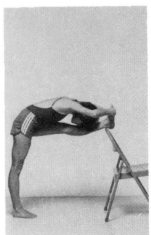

Scissor Stretch-Placement   Pose   Completed Pose

SITTING LEG STRETCHES

1. Placement. Sit in the the Stick Pose (see p. 169). Bend the right knee up and hold the ball of the foot with both hands. Sit tall!

2. Pose. Straighten the leg so foot is about eye level. Alternate between numbers one and two so that the leg pumps. Do 10 times or so.

3. Pose. When the leg has warmed up, bend the knee but bring it way back into the right armpit. This stretches the hip and upper hamstrings. Keep lifting the spine high. Do 5 to 10 times.

4. Pose. Begin with the knee under the right armpit as in No. 3. Place the right foot on the left upper arm, cradled above the left elbow. Place the right elbow around the right knee. Interlace the fingers. Keeping the right foot square, flat against the left arm, rock the leg back and forth. Stretch the hip, do not twist the knee.

Caution: If knees are painful discontinue until a teacher can be consulted.

Benefits: Stretches hamstrings, hips, knees. Strengthens arms and back.

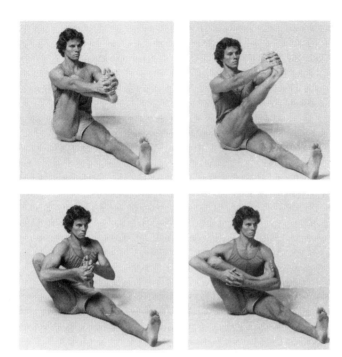

Left To Right From Top: Sitting Leg Stretch-Placement; Straighten
Leg; Knee Into Armpit; Leg Cradled.

THE ARCHER

(Akarna Dhanurasana)

1. Placement. Sit in Stick Pose (see p. 169). Hold the big toe of
each foot with the thumb and next two fingers of the corresponding hands. Do not let go of either toe through following
series.

2. Pose. Exhale, bend left knee up toward body, knee angles
out, elbow over knee. Right leg is straight and tight at the knee
throughout.

3. Pose. Exhale, straighten left leg out to side and hold for two
breaths. Bend it back as in No. 2.

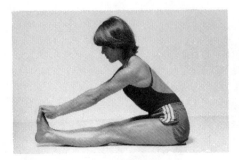

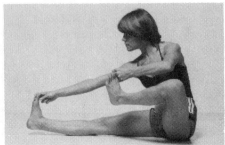

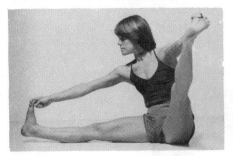

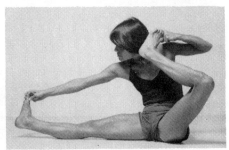

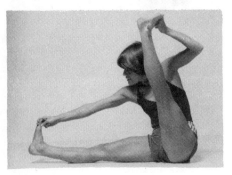

Left To Right From Top: The Archer-Placement; Knee Drawn Back; Knee Straightened; Foot to Ear; Straight Leg Drawn Up

4. Pose. Exhale, lift left foot up toward left ear. The knee goes back behind the left side. Bend knee and bring foot as in No. 2.

5. Pose. Exhale, lift left leg straight up as high as possible. The left elbow opens to the back. Hold, then bend the knee, straighten leg to Stick Pose, repeat on right leg. Do with each leg three or four times.

Benefits: Brings elasticity to legs, hips, lower spine. Strengthens arms, back. Relieves constipation.

BUTTERFLY HAMSTRING STRETCH

1. Placement. Lie on back, bend both knees into chest. Turn the backs of palms toward each other then hold each foot from the inner arch with respective hand. Keep shoulders and head on floor. Pelvis is in gentle dog tilt.

2. Pose. Exhale, lift right leg to ceiling, straightening as much as possible. Hold at maximum stretch just a second. Bend right knee, then repeat with left leg. Repeat as many as 20 times with each leg. On last stretch hold 10 seconds.

3. Pose. Exhale, let knees drop out to sides. Stretch right leg as far to right as possible. Hold at maximum stretch just a second. Bend right leg to original position. Reverse, taking left leg to far left. Repeat as many as 20 times with each leg. On last stretch hold 10 seconds.

4. Pose. Exhale, stretch both legs as far to sides as possible. Hold at maximum stretch just a second. Bend legs to original position. Build to 10 repetitions. Hold final stretch 10 to 15 seconds.

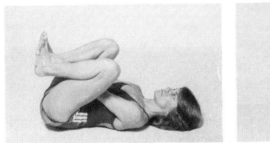
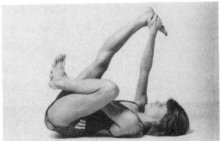
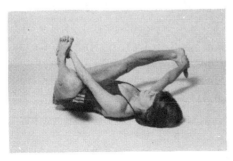
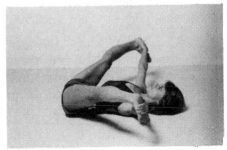

Left To Right From Top: Butterfly Stretch-Placement; Leg Straightened; Legs to Side; Butterfly Both Legs

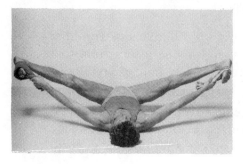

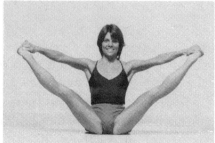

Butterfly Stretch with Towels   Seated Butterfly Stretch

5. Aid. If you can't hold feet and retain shoulders and head on ground wrap towels around balls of feet and hold ends of towels with hands. Proceed as described in Nos. 2, 3, 4.

6. Variation. Eventually, this pose is done while balancing on sitting bones. Don't be in any hurry to do this; it requires supple hamstrings and the back must be strong enough to sit without collapsing at the waist.

Benefits: Stretches hamstrings and adductors, strengthens hands and back.

RUNNER'S WARM-UP

1. Placement. Begin on all fours. Hands directly under shoulders, knees together. Place one foot on the floor in line with the other knee about 4 to 6 inches apart. Turn the toes of the back foot under toward knee.

2. Pose. Exhale, slowly straighten both legs, leaving hands and torso stretched down toward floor. To warm up the ankles, knees and hips, bend and then straighten legs several times. Finally, hold with straight legs, heels down for 10 to 15 seconds. Reverse.

3. Aid. This is very difficult in the beginning. To ease stretch, place yourself in front of a step, chair, or table. Place feet as described in No. 1. Place hands on ledge. Now follow directions for No. 2. Be sure to relax belly. Pelvis is in dog tilt.

Benefits: Warms up ankles, knees, hips; stretches legs.

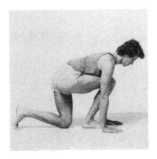
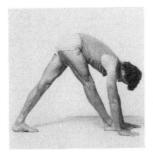
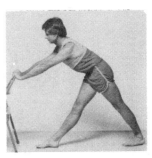

Runner's Warm-Up-Placement; Pose; With Chair

RECLINED SIDE STRETCH

(Anantasana)

1. Placement. Lie on your back in Mountain Pose. Roll over to your left side, rest on the left side. Bend the left arm to support your head with the left hand placed above the left ear. Left arm in line with extended, straight legs. Press out on balls of feet.

2. Pose. Exhale, bend right leg, grasp right big toe with right thumb and next two fingers. Exhale, extend right leg straight up. *Keep pelvic bones in a vertical plane.* Do cat tilt. Hold for 15 to 20 seconds. Lower leg, then head, roll over to right side, repeat.

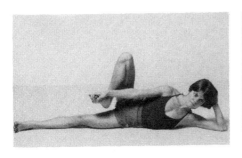
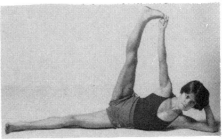

Reclined Side Stretch-Placement   Pose, Legs Extended

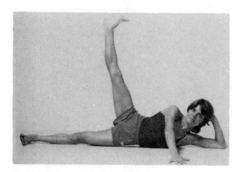 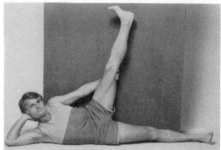

Reclined Side Stretch with Arm Support   Against Wall

3. Variation. Maintaining the stretch of the legs, the alignment of the body, and the balance is difficult in the beginning. Do No. 1 with the right hand on the floor in front of the chest. Then do No. 2 without holding the toe.

4. Aid. Do the pose with your back to the wall, beginning No. 1 with both buttocks 1 to 2 inches from wall. Eventually work with both buttocks touching the wall. Hold leg behind thigh, or with belt around foot if you can't hold the foot.

Benefits: Stretches hamstrings, helps strengthen and loosen pelvic area.

13

Relief: Back Stretches

There are two major areas a runner and other athletes should be stretching. The legs are clearly in need of effective stretching. But the area often ignored, which is a major site of misery, is the back.

Anatomically there are several salient facts relating to the back and running. Between the bones of the spine there are discs, hydraulic "shock absorbers," that allow for movement and compression. They account for the shape of the back and for one-fourth of its length. After the second decade of life, somewhere around twenty-five years of age, the arteries and the veins stop feeding into these disks. They then get their nutrition from the vertebrae and from their ability to imbibe from surrounding tissues. Therefore, the more movement in the back, the more opportunity the discs have to absorb nutrients and to maintain their hydraulic, elastic, and stress absorbing qualities.

Traversing the front and back of the spine, from top to bottom, are two long ligaments that support the spine. These ligaments keep the bones and the discs aligned by preventing excessive movement. Ligaments, like other connective tissues, contain micro-organs that contract but do not expand. So if these ligaments are not stretched, they stay contracted. When a person runs he is jumping vertically from foot to foot with over-all momentum downward due to gravity. The effect on the back, and particularly on the spinal disc, is one of compression. So, for the health of the back, stretching is essential to lengthen the ligaments encasing the discs. This lengthening will allow the discs to return to a more "plump," fuller state. Stretching creates more space between the vertebrae, thus deterring the flattening of the discs. Since there are no vacuums in the body, stretching the back allows for more intercellular fluid to bathe the discs, adding to their nutrition and health.

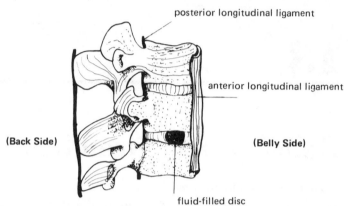

posterior longitudinal ligament

anterior longitudinal ligament

(Back Side)

(Belly Side)

fluid-filled disc

EVALUATING THE ELONGATION OF THE BACK

To stretch the back safely it must first be positioned correctly. As in forward bending the four natural curves of the back must be preserved. When stretching the back in a bent-over position, lift the buttocks in the dog tilt (see p. 26), pulling the kneecaps up. The entire torso must be straight so backbone moves as one unit. Then place one hand on the back of your waist. There should be a gentle indentation where the spine is. If the bones of the back poke up making bumps, then attempt to lift the buttocks higher. If the hamstrings are too tight this may not be possible. Then you must raise the torso until the vertebrae fall into the proper alignment. The belly must be relaxed.

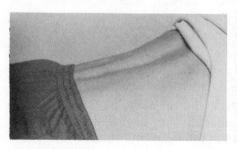

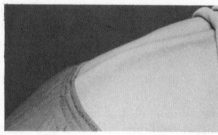

Correct Position of Spine for Back Stretches

Vertebrae Poking Out-**Incorrect** Position for Back Stretches

SINK STRETCH

1. Placement. Hold onto a sink, a window sill, or two knobs of an open door. Back away until you are bent at the hips, *not the waist,* forming an "L" shape. Keep the arms straight, and the head hanging naturally. Place hand on back to see if bones at back of waist poke out. If they do, do No. 3 below.

2. Pose. Another person holds your hips, and begins gently pulling backward. The assisting person protects his or her own back by keeping back flat, bending the knees. For greater leverage use a soft belt around the hips.

3. Variation. If your hamstrings are simply too tight to bring the back into proper alignment, eliminate the hamstrings by kneeling. Assisting person then squats with flat back, holds hips and leans back.

Benefits: Stretches the back, opens chest and shoulders, stretches hamstrings.

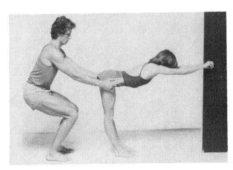
Sink Stretch-Pose Done Standing

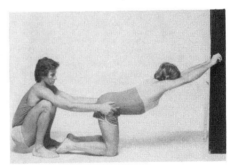
Variation for Tight Hamstrings

DOOR STRETCH

1. Placement. Tie the ends of a cloth belt together. Wrap it around the two knobs of an open door. Step inside the belt, your back to the door. Place the belt at the groin, rope taut. Keep feet parallel one foot apart, with kneecaps up. Place a chair in front of you.

2. Pose. Inhale, stretch arms overhead. Exhale, bend at the hips, where the belt is; lean away from the door and place the lower arms on the back of the chair. Touch the back of your waist to make sure vertebrae are in. Stretch into your fingertips. Hold for 20 to 30 seconds. Build to one to two minutes. As the hamstrings stretch, place arms on lower supports of chair, e.g., seat, lower rungs.

3. Variation. You can do this same stretch without the belt. Face a chair or ledge (maybe the top of the refrigerator), standing at an arm's length away. Feet are under hips. Place wrists on ledge, extend fingers outward, then on exhalation begin action of No. 2 by lifting buttocks to dog tilt. To eliminate stretch in hamstrings, you can kneel if necessary.

Benefits: Lengthens the spine, rejuvenates disks, opens chest and shoulders. Excellent way to learn correct forward bending.

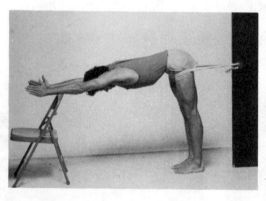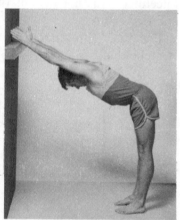

Left to Right: Door Stretch-Pose; Without Belt

FULL BODY STRETCH

1. Placement. Lie on back in Mountain Pose. Tuck pelvis firmly in cat tilt. Place arms overhead on floor, shoulders low, away from ears.

2. Pose. Without tensing the face, neck, or throat, stretch from heels to finger tips. Take care to keep feet squared by stretching the inside of the ankles and heels away from the body.

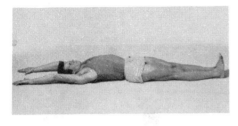

Full Body Stretch-Pose;

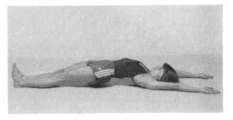

On Heels and Shoulders

3. Variation. Stretch one side at a time.

4. Variation. Press heels and shoulders into floor, squeeze buttocks, and lift entire torso off floor. Hold for a couple of breaths then place body back to floor.

Benefits: Stretches entire body, aligns spine.

Note: Use this pose between supine poses to realign the body. Excellent before or after Corpse Pose (see p. 200).

DOWNWARD DOG

(Adho Mukha Svanasana)

1. Placement. Kneel on all fours. Place hands and knees directly opposite each other, hands wide as shoulders and under your face, knees directly under the hips. Turn toes under. To avoid an uneven stretch in the feet, don't allow the heels to drop out, but keep heels above your toes. Lower shoulders away from ears.

2. Pose. Exhale and straighten knees. Stay high up on the toes and rotate the pelvis so buttock bones are turned toward ceiling. The pelvis is in dog tilt. Press with the hands and stretch bottom away from floor. Kneecaps pulled up. Relax the neck and stomach. With this alignment press heels down to floor. Hold 20 to 30 seconds. Release.

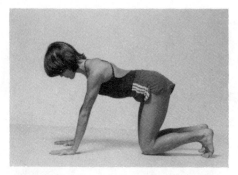
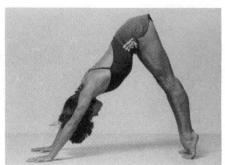
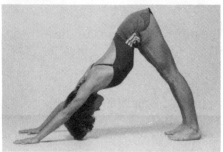

Clockwise From Top Left: Downward Dog-
Placement, Preparation on Toes; Completed
Pose, Heels Down

3. Variation. Beginner's Downward Dog on the Wall. Stand facing a wall; place palms opposite shoulders, fingers pointing up.
Walk feet back three feet or directly under your hips. Feet are a
foot apart, heels slightly wider than toes. Pull kneecaps up.

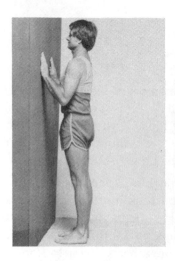
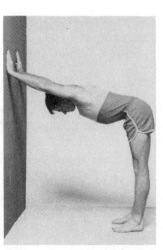

Beginner's Downward Dog-Preparation   Dog with Wall

Straighten arms, bring spine toward floor. Lift buttocks in dog tilt. Relax neck and belly. Walk into the wall to release.

4. Variation. When you can do No. 3 with no vertebrae poking up at the back of the waist, start moving down the wall. Kneel arm's length from chair braced against wall. Curl toes under, straighten legs. Stay up on toes as you rotate bottom up toward ceiling. Lower back should be flat, with no vertebrae poking up. Keep lifting hips; stretch heels back to the floor. Relax neck and stomach. Hold 30 seconds.

5. Aid. When you can do No. 4 with no vertebrae poking up on the lower back you are ready to do Downward Dog on the Floor. Kneel on all fours. Place the thumb and index finger of each hand into the base of a wall, curb, or step. Follow directions for No. 1 and No. 2. Press equally on the inside and outside of the hand.

Benefits: This is the perfect pose for running athletes. It stretches the entire back side of the body, the soles of the feet, the Achilles tendon. It strengthens and relieves tension in the upper

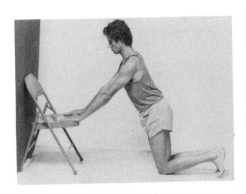

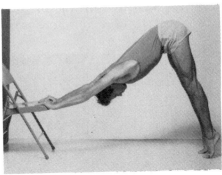

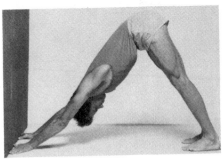

Clockwise From Top Left: Downward Dog With Chair-Preparation; Buttocks High, On Toes; Heels Down

body. It opens the chest and improves breathing. It is excellent both before and after running.

HANGING

1.   Pose. To stretch the upper back, hang from the arms. Not only does the back benefit but this is an excellent way to stretch wrists, elbows, shoulders. Good for baseball players, tennis players, etc.

2. Pose. To stretch lower back, hang from knees. Place bar in doorway at about neck level. Place hands on the floor, nearly under the bar. Bend one leg. Exhale, kick off with other leg. Do handstand and bend both knees over bar. Hold opposite elbows allowing arms and body to hang. Relax and lengthen. To intensify stretch, place weighted objects under you; hold them in your hands. Hold pose as long as you can. Place hands on floor. Kick one leg down at a time.

Benefits: Instead of gravity working to compress the spine as it usually does, this pose uses gravity to open the spine.

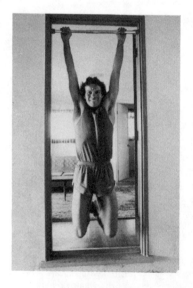
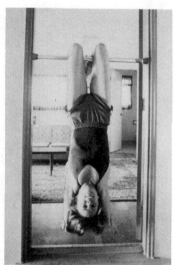

Hanging Back Stretch-From Hands   From Knees

KNEES TO CHEST

(Apanasana)

1. Placement. Lie on back in Mountain Pose. Bend the knees and drag the heels up to buttocks. Exhale, bend knees over chest, interlace fingers below knees.

2. Pose. Exhale, push heels away from body, squeeze knees into chest and relax stomach. Lengthen neck but do not tense it. Do gentle dog tilt.

3. Variation. To decrease stretch, place hands on thighs under knees. Squeeze knees in; on exhalation lift forehead to knees. Hold 5 to 10 seconds, release. This is excellent to do after Shoulder Stand (see p. 156). It releases tension in the lower back and neck.

4. Variation. Increase stretch by interlacing fingers behind balls of feet. Lift head to knees on exhalation. Inhale as you release.

Benefits: Stretches entire back, particularly lower back. Classic wind relieving pose.

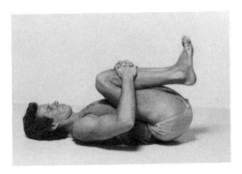
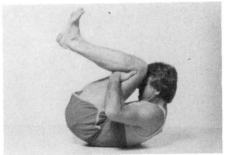
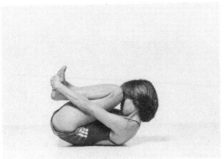

Clockwise From Top Left: Knees to Chest-Pose with Hands on Lower Legs; Hands Under Knees Head Up; Hands Wrapped Around Feet

SPINAL ROLL

1. Placement. Sit on well-padded mat. Interlace your fingers behind your knees which are bent, feet on floor. Place forehead on or near knees.

2. Pose. Keep body in this position and on an exhalation slowly lean back. Gently rock back and forth between buttocks and shoulders. Allow the legs to create a free-swinging momentum.

3. Variation. After rolling back and forth 10 or more times rest on shoulders and upper back, hold with knees on forehead. Exhale, roll to sitting.

4. Variation. After your back has gained some flexibility hold No. 3 above. On exhalation straighten one leg and hold for 10 seconds. Reverse legs. Then on exhalation straighten both legs so tips of toes are on ground overhead. Hold 10 seconds, bend knees, slowly roll down.

Benefits: Gentle warm-up for back and legs. Also, good to relieve tension in back.

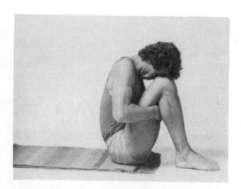

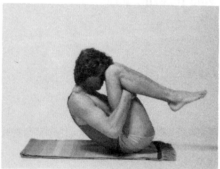

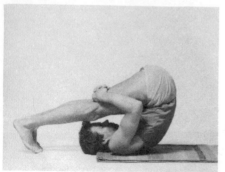

Clockwise From Top Left: Spinal Roll-Placement; Pose Done Rolling; Hold on Shoulders

CROSSED–LEG SPINAL ROLL

1. Placement. Sit on a well-padded mat with your legs crossed at the ankles. Hold the top of your left foot with your right hand. Hold the top of the right foot with the left hand. Legs are crossed, arms are not.

2. Pose. Inhale, sit tall. Exhale, round the back and place your forehead to the floor or as near to it as possible. Maintain this "ball" position with the body and inhale as you roll backward on the spine until you are high up on the shoulders. Exhale, roll back to sitting. Then repeat by inhaling to sit tall, exhale head to floor and so on.

3. Variation. Do the above 6 to 10 times. When back is loose do the above but straighten the legs as much as possible and place toes on floor when you have rolled to your shoulders. Bend knees to roll up. Be sure to reverse this entire series by crossing your legs so the opposite leg is on the bottom when sitting.

Benefits: Develops coordination and balance. Warms up and stretches back.

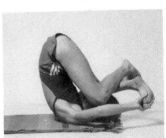
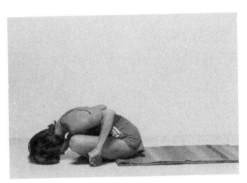
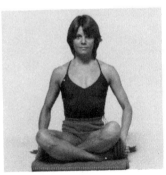
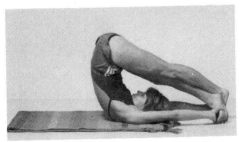

Left to Right From Top: Crossed-Leg Spiral Roll-Preparation; Head to Floor; Roll to Shoulders; Straighten Legs

14

Suspension: Standing Forward Bends

Most people think that bending over to touch their toes indicates the degree of flexibility in the back of their legs. This is because the hamstrings are such "screamers" that this is where you feel the stretch. In fact, much of this forward bend comes from the back.

The hamstring (back of thigh) muscles begin at the buttocks bones and connect below the knees. The only way to stretch these muscles fully is to straighten the knees and bend *from the hips* as though suspended from the sitting bones. The way most people touch their toes is to bend from the waist. (Stand up and try it both ways.) Continual stretching in this way misaligns the body and is dangerous to the back.

Many of us have rounded backs because almost everything we do is forward, to the front of us. Continual stretching with a rounded back reinforces this tendency. But remember that there are two long ligaments that support the spine from top to bottom. One ligament supports the outer, back side of the spine and the other ligament supports the front, belly side of the spine. When rounding your back to touch your toes, the outer ligament stretches but the front one, the one on the belly side, contracts. Unless this imbalance is counteracted the ligaments of the back become uneven in length causing the back to curve forward more. The strength of the back dissipates.

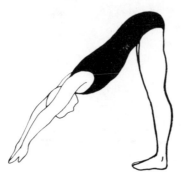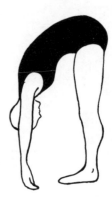

Correct bending from the hips   Incorrect bending from the waist

Further, the hamstring muscles are usually stronger than the back. If you start tugging on the two simultaneously and there is a weak spot, injury is more likely to occur in the back. Stretching this way puts tremendous pressure on the spinal discs because the angle between the inner edge of the vertebrae decreases, forcing the nucleus of the discs backward. All of this can easily be avoided by learning to forward bend correctly. Here is the most important principle: *When bending forward either standing or sitting, consider the back a single unit and bend from the hips.* To do this the pelvis must be in the dog tilt, with the buttocks stretching away from the knees.

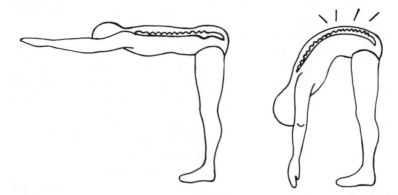

Bending from HIPS promotes correct spinal alignment; bending from WAIST leads to spinal misalignment.

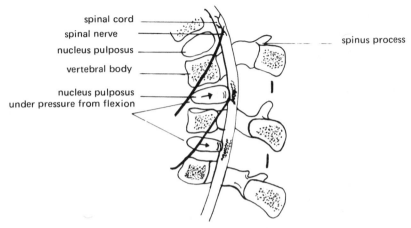

spinal cord

spinal nerve

nucleus pulposus

vertebral body

nucleus pulposus
under pressure from flexion

spinus process

**Resulting pressure on discs from
improper forward bending**

This strengthens and protects the back. When tilting the pelvis forward the back muscles must be contracted and strengthened to prevent the back from rounding and giving into gravity. When the back is one unit, "straight," no one curve of the back is curving against its natural angle, so the discs and vertebrae are not forced out of alignment.

Before beginning these poses read the preliminary instructions for back stretches (see p. 121). On page 122 there are instructions for evaluating the elongation of the back. Apply this test to all standing forward bends at the horizontal position. This insures that the back is lengthened, stretched before bending it. When bending forward to place the stomach on the thighs the bones of the back will probably poke out.

WALL HANG

1. Placement. Stand with back against a wall; place feet 8 inches from wall, 8 inches apart. Heels are slightly wider than toes. Draw kneecaps up by contracting the quadriceps. Do cat tilt and place entire spine (except the neck) on the wall. Place hands on groin. This is where you will bend.

2. Preliminary Movement. Exhale, treat the entire spine as one unit; bring top of head away from wall. Buttocks lift in dog tilt;

they move up the wall. Front of body is as open as back. Touch spine at back of waist. There should be an indentation, a trough running up the back at the bones of the spine. If the bones poke up above the muscles, then lift the entire torso higher in order to keep bones in.

3. Pose. Now allow the back to round down very gently, aiming the top of the head to the feet, *not* to the knees. Arms and head hang. If hands touch floor, hold each elbow. Feel gravity pull; relax stomach; allow muscles and ligaments of back to lengthen. Hold 15 seconds, build time to one minute. To come out of pose, tuck buttom down and roll back up the wall.

4. Variation. Do No. 3 holding each elbow with opposite hand. Lift the elbows out toward the center of the room. With each breath stretch the armpits toward the floor; this lengthens the

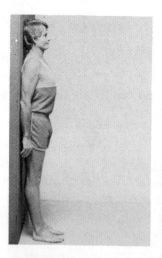
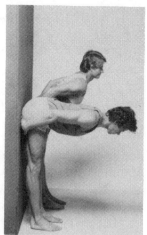

Clockwise From Top Left: Wall Hang-Placement; Preliminary Movement; Hanging Pose; Holding Elbows; Lifted Elbows

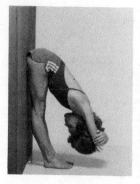
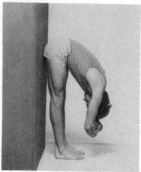
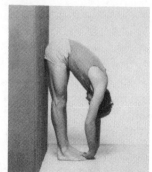

spine. To release, drop arms down, tuck pelvis into cat tilt and roll back up the wall.

Benefits: This is a marvelous way to learn proper forward bending because you should feel buttocks move up the wall. The back legs are given wonderful stretch.

SPREAD FOOT FORWARD BEND

(Prasarita Padottanasana)

1. Placement. Begin in Mountain Pose. Jump the feet 5 feet apart. Feet parallel, kneecaps drawn up. Place hands at the groins.

2. Pose. Exhale; treat the spine as one unit, bend forward from the hip sockets. Exhale. Place the hands on the floor, wide as the shoulders in line, with the feet. Inhale, lift the head and the buttocks, lengthen the back. Relax the stomach. Exhale, bend the elbows back between the knees and place the head on the floor. Elbows form right angles. Hold twenty seconds. To release, reverse procedure, straightening elbows first, lifting back as unit.

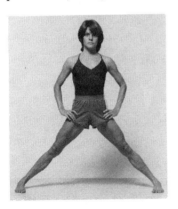 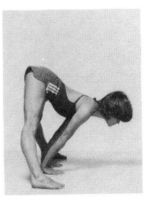 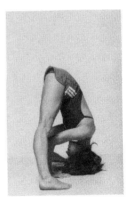

Spread Foot Forward   Hands on Floor   Pose
Bend-Placement

3. Aid. Place a chair 2½ feet in front of you. Follow the same directions as in No. 2, except place hands on the seat of the chair rather than the floor. If the back bones of the waist still poke up, place hands on back of chair. To release, tuck pelvis down into cat tilt, then round the back up, one vertebra at a time.

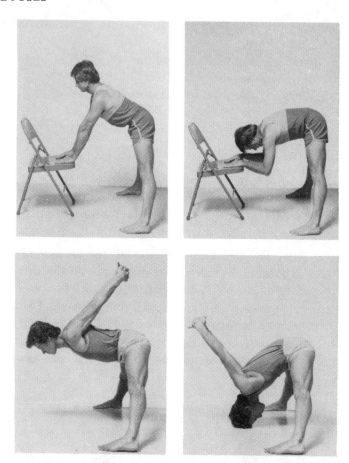

Left to Right from Top: Spread Foot Forward Bend-Hands on Chair, Back Straight; Pose with Chair; Fingers Interlaced, Torso Horizontal; Top of Head to Floor

4. Variation. Interlace fingers behind the buttocks, open chest. Exhale, bend at hips and bring torso as far forward as possible with back flat. Lift arms away from buttocks. Exhale, extend the top of the head toward floor, bring arms as far over head as possible. Hold 15 to 20 seconds. Inhale, lift to standing. If you can't interlace fingers behind you, hold pole or cloth. Slowly work hands together.

Benefits: Stretches hamstrings, inner thighs, back. Strengthens legs, ankles. Excellent for upper body tension. Variation 4 stretches chest, shoulders, and arms.

STANDING TOE HOLDING POSE

(Padangusthasana)

1. Placement. Stand, feet 1 foot apart. Kneecaps up tightly.

2. Pose. Exhale, bend forward from the hips and grasp big toes with first two fingers and thumbs; palms face each other. Straighten the arms, lift the head and lift the buttocks high in dog tilt. Lower shoulders away from the ears. Relax the stomach!! Exhale, bend the elbows out to sides and lengthen the spine toward the floor so the head comes to shins. Hold 10 seconds. Release by straightening arms, then stand up on inhalation.

3. Aid. Place a belt or rope under the arches of the feet. Exhale, bend over, then grasp the ends of the rope. Straighten the legs and arms. Do dog tilt. Look up and lift the torso high enough to draw the bones at the back of the waist in. Keep extending the back. Exhale, bend the elbows out and lengthen the top of the head toward the floor. Hold 2 breaths. Drop the rope, tuck the pelvis in cat tilt and roll the spine to standing.

Benefits: Stretches legs and back.

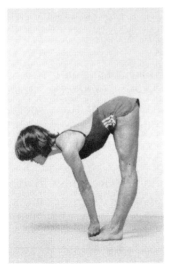

Standing Toe Holding Pose
-Head and Buttocks Lifted

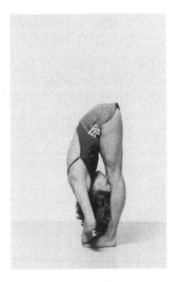

Head to Shins

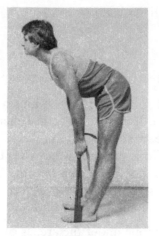

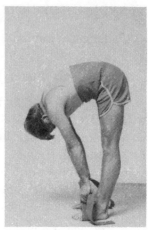

Toe Holding Pose with Belt   Completed Pose
-Head and Buttocks Lifting

STANDING, INTENSE STRETCH OF THE BACK

(Uttanasana)

1. Placement. Stand in Mountain Pose, kneecaps up.

2. Pose. Inhale; lift arms over head. Keep shoulders away from ears throughout. Exhale; bend at the hips; place hands on the floor beside the feet. Lift head and buttocks. Pelvis is in dog tilt. Move the weight forward onto the balls of the feet distributing weight over entire foot. Exhale; lower head to shins. Relax the stomach. Hold 2 breaths, build to a minute. Inhale; lift head; inhale; lift torso as one unit.

3. Aid. If your hands don't touch the floor, place books by the sides of your feet as shown. Place hands on these, fingers pointing forward, and proceed as in No. 2. Be sure kneecaps are pulled up. Hips in dog tilt.

4. Variation. To increase stretch, begin in No. 2, move the hands further back behind the feet, fingers point forward and parallel. Legs are vertical. Keep lifting buttocks. Soften the back

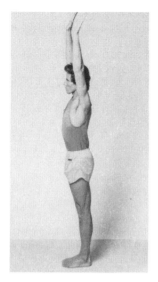 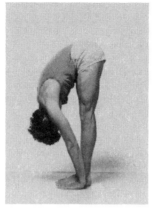 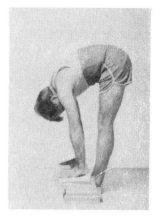

From Left: Standing, Intense Stretch of Back-Arms Overhead; Hands Next to Feet; Hands on Books

of the legs and under the buttock bones. Arms are straight. Relax neck and stomach. As body gains flexibility palms will be on floor.

5. Variation. To intensify stretch, place the right forearm on the right calf, the left forearm on the left calf. Soften the neck and stomach. Move the shoulders toward the waist. Exhale, draw the entire spine toward the legs. Breathe and hold 5 seconds, increase to 30 seconds.

Benefits: Stretches entire back side of the body.

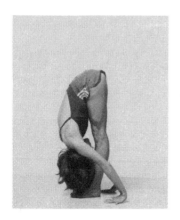 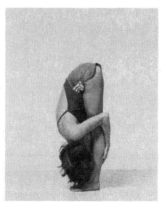

Hands Behind Feet   Lower Arms on Calves

15

Breathe Again: Backbending

Backbending brings life to the spine, opens the chest, and stretches the entire front side of the body. Only the most basic poses are given here, but even with these you can experience the exhilarating energy they bring. The increased mobility from backbending brings a greater blood supply to the discs and the nerves of the spinal cord. With backbending the rib cage expands, increasing the quantity and quality of the breath. Any athlete who has breathing problems can benefit from these poses. Finally, the musculature on the front of the body stretches, as well as the knees, thighs, groins, stomach, and chest.

There are some important principles of backbending. *Before arching the back, lengthen the back.* Do a couple of the poses described in Chapter 8, the Sink Stretch, Downward Dog. When backbending do not attempt to bring the tailbone to the head. *Always tuck the tailbone into the body firmly, it extends downward in the cat tilt.* Never hold a backbending position longer than the buttocks can contract. Soften the stomach! *Do not tense the neck.*

Before doing any backbending poses, strengthen the muscles of the back by doing the Locust (see p. 144) and Preparation for Cobra (see p. 145) frequently for one or two months. Thereafter, do these at least twice a week.

If you should get a headache when backbending it probably means you are over arching and/or tensing the neck while doing these poses. The neck should always be relaxed and as long as possible. When doing the poses beginning in a prone position lift the head but keep the chin in toward the chest. The back of the neck should be long.

Caution: If you have high blood pressure consult a teacher before doing these stretches.

PRONE BACK STRETCH

Pose. First lengthen the back by lying face down. Stretch the arms overhead on the floor, point the toes, keep inner edges of the legs together. Stretch, lengthen from fingertips to toes.

Benefits: Easy back stretch.

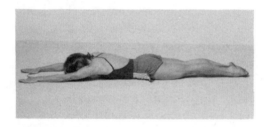

Prone Back Stretch-Pose

LOCUST

(Salabhasana)

1. Placement. Lie face down on a protected surface. Place the front of the chin on the floor. Keep toes pointed, inner ankles and knees touching. Palms on floor next to hips.

2. Pose. Maintain contact with the floor with both hips and on exhalation lift the right leg straight up. The knees face the floor. Soften throat and neck. Hold for three breaths. Release on exhalation. Realign the body, repeat with left leg. As strength increases build up length of holds.

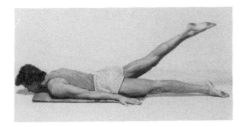

Locust-Single Leg Lift

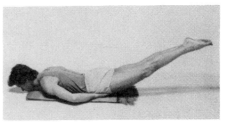

Both Legs Lifted

3. Pose. To do with both legs, turn hands to face body and place the knuckles opposite the groin (the crease where the leg attaches to the body). Exhale, lift both legs up, feet together and knees straight. Hold for three breaths at first. People with weak backs should do one leg for at least a month before attempting two legs.

Benefits: By lifting against gravity these poses strengthen the muscles of the lower back. Muscle tone here is essential for posture, and basic to all further development.

PREPARATION FOR COBRA

(Bhujangasana)

1. Placement. Lie face down on protected surface. Forehead on floor, arms to sides, palms in, inner edges of legs and feet together, toes pointed.

2. Pose. Keep feet on floor; inhale and lift the head and upper chest as high as possible. Hands reach back toward feet. *Look forward or down slightly.* Hold for three breaths; increase time.

3. Variation. Do the same action but change the arms. First stretch arms straight out from shoulders. Last, place arms on floor overhead. In all three of these variations it is important that the breath flow. This may cause the torso to rock slightly. Holding the breath may lift you a fraction higher but will drain you of strength.

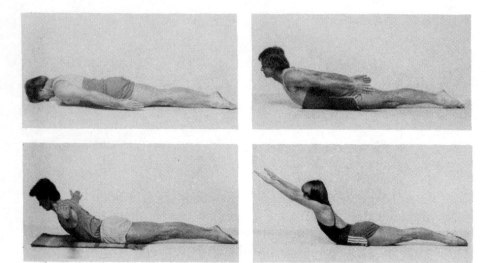

Left to Right From Top: Placement; Pose with Hands Back; Hands to Sides; Hands Overhead

Benefits: This pose strengthens the upper back muscles. Anyone who tends to have rounded shoulders should do these variations frequently—at least two or three times a week.

SUPPORTED CHEST OPENER

1. Placement. Sit sideways on a sofa that has rounded arm support. Position yourself so when you lie back your head is supported and your chest is open.

2. Pose. Lower your shoulder blades, softening shoulders away from the ears. Palms face up, keep opening the armpits upward. Tuck pelvis in cat tilt. With each inhalation lift the breast bone higher and higher.

3. Variation. To increase stretch lift both arms overhead and stretch into fingertips. Do not tense neck and face muscles. Once this gets comfortable, hold weighted object such as a book in the hands.

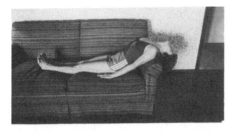
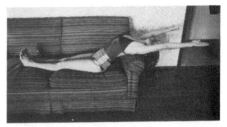
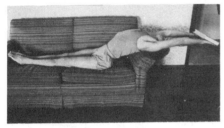
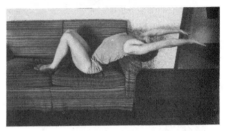

Left to Right From Top: Supported Chest Opener-Pose; Arms Overhead; Holding Weight; Knees Bent to Protect Back

Two cautions: If your lower back should complain bend your knees, place feet on the sofa. If you carry your head forward you may not be able to do this and could benefit tremendously by working with a teacher.

Benefits: Stretches upper chest.

BRIDGE POSE

(Setu Banda)

1. Placement. Lie on back. Roll shoulders back and down, palms down. Face is directed to ceiling. Bend knees, place feet parallel to each other, close to outside of buttocks. *Knees above toes.*

2. Pose. Exhale, squeeze buttocks and lift one vertebra at a time, beginning with tailbone. *Pelvis is tucked in cat tilt.* Press on inside of feet and lift entire spine. Hold 20 to 30 seconds. Roll down from upper back.

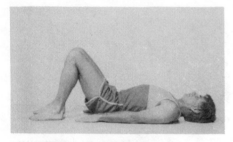
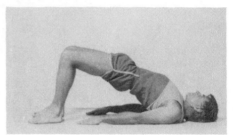
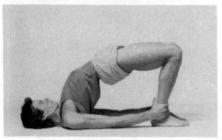

From Top Left: Bridge Pose-Placement; Pose;
Holding Ankles

3. Variation. To increase leverage begin in No. 1 but hold each ankle with corresponding hand. Proceed as in No. 2, pull with arms to open chest. Relax face and neck.

Benefits: Besides the many benefits listed before on backbending, this pose works to stretch and strengthen the knees. It also is excellent for opening the upper chest.

CAMEL POSE

(Ustrasana)

1. Placement. Kneel, with legs four to six inches apart, front of foot on floor. Hand on hips. Lower shoulders and lift chest high, not forward.

2. Pose. Contract the buttocks in strong cat tilt of the pelvis. Arch the back and extend the chest. Keeping pelvis pushed forward, exhale, place one hand at a time on the heels, or sole of each foot. Allow the head to drop back. Hold for two breaths. Build to 20 to 30 seconds.

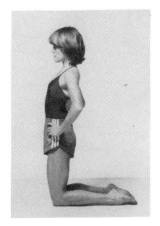
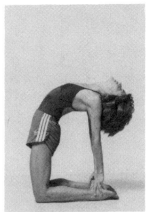
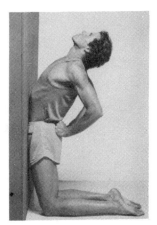

| Camel Pose-Placement | Pose | Against Wall |

3. Variation. Beginners should kneel three inches from wall. Place fists on upper buttocks, palms in, elbows parallel. Cat tilt, pubis moves toward wall. Draw the chest up. Exhale, drop head back. Keep lifting and arch slightly.

Cautions: *People with neck problems should not do this pose without a teacher.*

Benefits: If you have rounded shoulders, do this pose often. It tones entire spine.

UPWARD DOG

(Urdhva Mukha Svanasana)

1. Placement. Lie face down. Hands next to chest, middle fingers parallel to each other. Elbows are in, not hanging out to sides. Feet are a foot apart. Toes pointed back. Do cat tilt, pull kneecaps up firmly.

2. Pose. Inhale, straighten the arms, lift the chest, look forward or very slightly up. The body is supported on hands and front of the feet only, the *pubis is off the floor.* Arch the back by drawing the spine forward with *buttocks tight,* knees pulled up. The

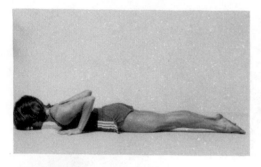

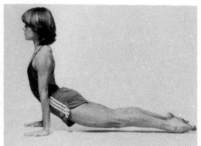

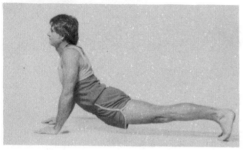

From Top Left: Upward Dog-Placment;
Pose on Front of Feet; Pose on Toes

shoulders are away from the ears. Hold for two breaths. Build up to 10 to 15 seconds.

3. Beginners. Do the exact same pose but keep the toes turned under. Lower the shoulders away from the ears.

Benefits: This pose brings elasticity to the spine. It can be very helpful in relieving back pain. It brings blood to the pelvic region.

BOW

(Dhanurasana)

1. Placement. Lie face down. Lengthen the body, inner edges of legs and feet touching. Exhale, bring the heels to the buttocks. Knees may separate but *keep legs parallel.* Reach back with the arms and hold the right ankle with the right hand; hold left ankle with left hand.

2. Pose. Exhale, lift and pull the legs away from the head as though reaching for the ceiling with your feet. The thighs and

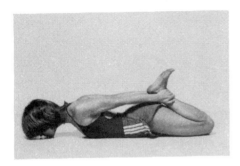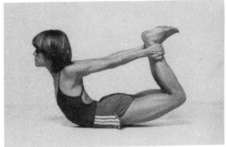

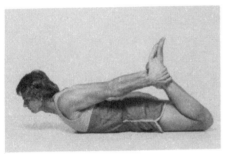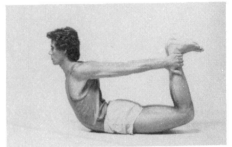

Left to Right From Top: Bow-Placement; Pose with Feet Lifting; Groin Stretch to Floor, Feet Pulled Back

chest lift from the floor. The arms are straight. *Squeeze the buttocks.* Look very slightly up. Breathe and hold for 15 seconds.

3. Variation. Begin in No. 1. Exhale; squeeze the buttocks and flatten the front of the groin into the floor. Hold two breaths. Work up to 20 seconds to one minute. Do this slowly so the knees are not inadvertently over-stretched. This is an excellent stretch for the groin area.

4. Variation. Begin in No. 1. Exhale, *squeeze the buttocks.* Inhale, leave knees on the floor and pull feet away from head. Head and chest lift high off the floor. Soften stomach, relax neck, look straight ahead. Lower shoulders. Hold 2 breaths, build to 30 seconds.

Benefits: Brings elasticity and strength to the spine. Stretches the groins.

16

Topsy Turvy: Inverted Poses

Because gravity is a constant force few of us realize its incredible hold over us. But whether we are consciously aware of it or not we certainly can see the effects of gravity by looking at a random group of people. The power of gravity is reflected in sagging faces, breasts, bellies, and spines. The bones themselves are often misshapen by the compensations made in the effort to stay upright.

The yogis have dealt with this problem for literally centuries. Rather than ignoring the seemingly insurmountable problem they have put gravity to good use by simply inverting the body for some time every day. When the body is turned upside down the inner organs reverse their course. Also, the body fluids are stimulated to move. As this happens there is a greater exchange of fluids in each cell, nutrients are absorbed, wastes are discarded. With gravity's help the brain is flushed; the pituitary gland in the head, and thyroid and parathyroid glands in the neck are bathed with a fresh supply of blood. The venous blood in the lower body flows freely toward the heart. Elimination is stimulated.

Elevating the legs after exercise is extremely important. Any running activity concentrates the flow of blood in the lower limbs. Unless this is reversed the legs sometimes feel heavy, the brain and heart sluggish. The Shoulder Stand, or any of its variations, can remedy these effects in minutes. This pose can be particularly beneficial if you work out in the morning and then sit or stand most of the day.

In the first pose, the Shoulder Stand, the musculation of the arms, shoulders, neck are strengthened. In addition the lower back, belly and leg muscles are toned by the essential work of balancing upside down. This pose is one of total equilibrium. The entire body must coordinate its efforts to do the pose properly.

Although you may not believe it at first, the Shoulder Stand has a soothing effect on the nerves and acts to bring about relaxation. If you run or work out at night and find that this stimulates you to wakefulness, needed sleep will be more accessible after a five to ten minute shoulder stand. But no matter when you choose to do this pose be sure to include it in your yoga practice or fitness routine. Soon, you won't have to be told about the benefits of inverting the body; they will be yours.

Because the vertebrae of the neck are much smaller than the rest of the spine they are not designed to hold a lot of weight. To prevent this, do not press the back of the neck into the floor. This is a *shoulder* stand, not a neck stand. To preserve the concave curve of the neck most of us need to work with our shoulders raised slightly higher than the back of the head. To do this place a folded blanket, about one or two inches thick, under your shoulders and arms. The back of the head is on the floor, the back of the neck is still in its natural concave curve, gently arching into the body.

In the Shoulder Stand the back of the neck will be lengthening so expect the feeling of stretch. If the neck complains, very gently lift the chin a half inch or so, relax the neck, throat, face. Or, you might lift the shoulders still higher by placing a second or even third blanket under them. However, if you feel strain in the neck, stop for awhile and try again later after practicing more standing poses. If you still have problems, consult a teacher. *To protect the neck never turn the head from side to side in the Shoulder Stand or Plough.*

Frequently in the beginning there will be discomfort in the lower back and neck after doing these inverted poses. For relief, do the Knee to Chest Pose, Variation 3 (p.110). Lift the head to the knees 3 or 4 times or until discomfort is gone.

Caution: People with high blood pressure should not do these poses without a trained teacher.

For Women: During the menstrual period do not invert the body.

NECK STRETCH

1. Placement. Lie on back in Mountain Pose. Bend knees and place feet on floor below each buttock. Interlace fingers behind head.

2. Pose. Exhale, and with the neck and head completely passive, lift the head with the hands. Bring the head as far forward as possible without strain. Shoulders are low, away from the ears.

Benefits: Stretches and relieves tension in neck and upper shoulders. Prepares for Shoulder Stand and Plough.

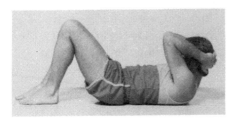

Neck Stretch-Pose, Head Passive

HARE POSE

1. Placement. Sit on heels, feet parallel as in Preparation for Hero's Pose (see p. 81). Place palms on floor next to knees. Round your back, tuck your chin in toward chest and place top of head on floor in front of knees.

2. Pose. Exhale, lift buttocks and roll toward back of head. Shoulders must be low, away from ears. Distribute weight among head, hands and knees. Hold 10 to 15 seconds; build time.

Benefits: Excellent for upper shoulder tension, headaches. Prepares for inverted poses.

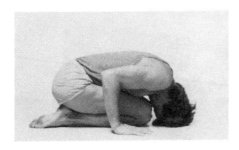
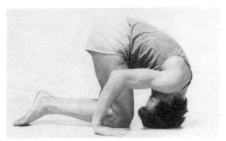

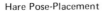

Hare Pose-Placement   Pose

SHOULDER STAND

(Salamba Sarvangasana)

1. Placement. Lie on the floor in the Mountain Pose. Place a folded blanket under the torso only. Roll the shoulders toward the floor, open the chest. Palms down. *Never turn the head in this pose.* Exhale; bend the knees over the chest.

2. Pose. Exhale, press the hands into the floor, contract the stomach and lift the buttocks toward the ceiling. Bend elbows and place palms on back as close to floor as possible. Fingers point toward each other. Exhale; lift knees toward ceiling. Pelvis is in cat tilt. Exhale, straighten legs. Inner feet and legs touch. Tighten kneecaps. Entire body lifts toward ceiling. Press balls of feet

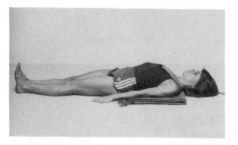
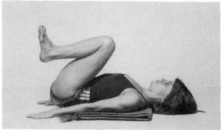
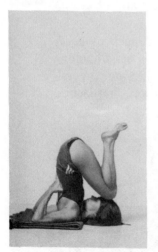
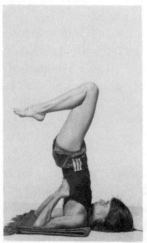
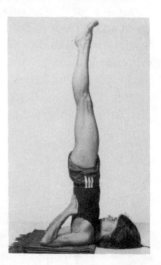

Left to Right From Top: Shoulder Stand-Placement with Mat under Torso; Knees to Chest; On Shoulders, Knees to Head; Knees Lifted; Completed Pose

toward ceiling. Allow the neck, face and throat to be passive. Hold 20 to 30 seconds, build to 5 minutes. To release, bend knees to head, place hands to floor, slowly roll the back to the floor. The head remains on the floor throughout.

3. Variation. In the beginning you may not have the flexibility to lift high, onto the top of the shoulders. Place the hands on the back closer to the buttocks. The legs will be at an angle, over the head. As flexibility and strength increase, work toward lifting the body until it is perpendicular to the floor.

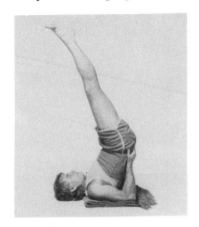

Half Shoulder Stand

4. Aid. Lie with your buttocks against a wall, stretch the legs up the wall (see Stick Pose, p. 169). Bend your knees and place feet on wall. Exhale and press feet into wall; beginning with the tailbone lift one vertebra at a time until you are on top of shoulders and back of head. Interlace fingers and stretch hands toward the wall and down to the floor. Keeping elbows close to each other, release your hands and place them on your back as close to the floor as possible. Do the above every day for a week, then lift one foot from the wall. Place that foot back to the wall, then lift the other. Do this every day for a week. With this type of cautious preparation you are now ready to take both feet off the wall. Do so one leg at a time. Spine comes into body and lifts toward ceiling. Align knees and feet so they are straight. Hold 15 to 20 seconds. To come down, place one foot at a time back against wall; roll down slowly.

Benefits: Relieves fatigue, calms and rejuvenates body, strengthens upper body, stretches neck.

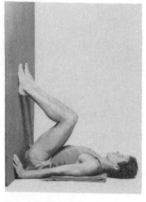 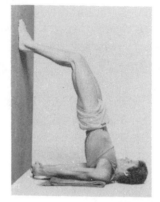 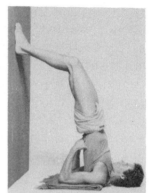

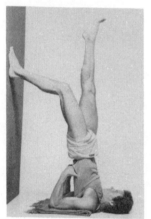 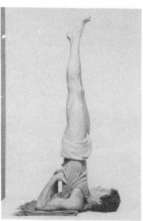

Left to Right From Top:
Shoulder Stand With Wall;
Feet on Wall; Torso Lifted;
Hands on Back; One Leg
Extended; Pose

THE PLOUGH

(Halasana)

1. Placement. Begin in Shoulder Stand (see p. 156).

2. Pose. Exhale, lower the legs overhead until the tips of the toes touch the floor. Keep feet perpendicular to floor. The pelvis is now in the dog tilt which enables the back to be long and straight, not rounded. Keep stretching the pubis away from the nose. The knees are tight, the face, neck and stomach are passive. Hold 10 to 15 seconds. Increase time slowly to 1 to 2 minutes. To release, place hands on floor and roll one vertebra at a time to the floor.

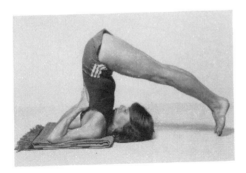

Plough-Completed Pose

3. Aid. Lie on your back with the top of your head toward a wall. Stretch your arms overhead and place yourself so fingers are 1 or 2 inches away from wall. Then lower arms to sides. Do the Shoulder Stand with hands on back. To do Plough, exhale, and lower both legs overhead until feet are on wall. If hamstrings are short the legs will be higher up the wall. The bones of the back waist should be slightly indented, not poking out. If hamstrings are longer the legs will be horizontal or even closer to the floor. No matter where your feet are, push with hands and feet, and lift sitting bones higher. Relax face, neck and belly.

4. Variation. Do the Plough and interlace fingers behind you. Straighten arms and stretch them down to floor and away from body. This opens chest and stretches shoulders and arms.

5. Aid. If your arms, shoulders and/or chest are tight you may not be able to interlace fingers behind you. In that case hold a pole or towel in your hands, straighten arms and stretch them

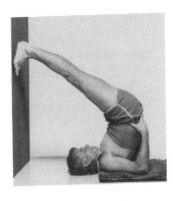

Plough with Wall

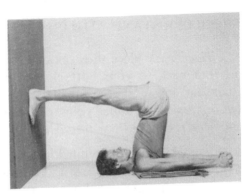

Interlaced Fingers Stretched Away from Body

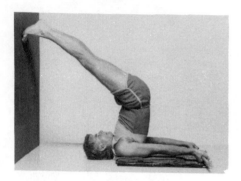

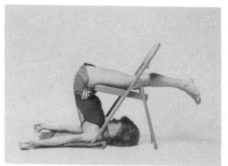

Plough Holding Pole   Plough with Chair Support

down to floor. As flexibility increases, walk your hands closer and closer to each other. Discard aid when hands touch.

6. Aid. The Plough, when done over a chair, is a marvelous resting pose. It is also helpful in relieving headaches. Lie in Mountain Pose and place a hardback chair at your head. Lift to Shoulder Stand with knees bent, then straighten legs out on chair. Pull chair into groin. Relax. The arms are on the floor. Once this gets comfortable, hold as long as you like.

Benefits: Same as Shoulder Stand, but also stretches legs and strengthens back.

SHOULDER STAND WITH CHAIRS

1. Placement. Place the back of a sturdy chair against a wall. Lie on your back so your buttocks are in line with the edge of the chair seat, lower legs are on the seat. Be sure to use a mat, one or two inches thick, under your torso only. The head is on the floor, and *neck is off the floor throughout.*

2. Preparation. Bend your knees and place the feet on the edge of the seat. Exhale, squeeze the buttocks and lift the torso high. Interlace your fingers behind you and stretch them down to the floor and back toward the wall. Squeeze the shoulder blades and

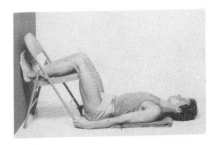

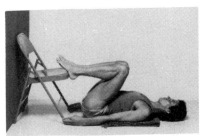

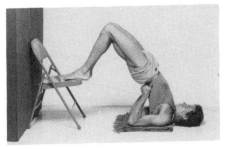

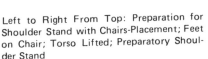

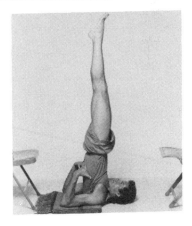

Left to Right From Top: Preparation for
Shoulder Stand with Chairs-Placement; Feet
on Chair; Torso Lifted; Preparatory Shoulder Stand

stretch the chest. Relax the neck, throat and face. Place your
hands on your back.

3. Preparation. Exhale, lift one leg up to ceiling, then exhale,
lift the other. Hold for a few breaths in Shoulder Stand.

4. Preparation. Exhale, bend at the hips and lower the legs to
a chair placed behind your head, arm's length away. Do a Plough
(see p. 158). (If you are very stretched you *may* not need the
second chair.) Secured in this fashion, release your hands and hold
the legs of the chair at your back. Pull the chair in until it touches
your back.

5. Pose. With your upper arms inside the front legs of the chair,
hold the back legs up at the seat. Use this as a lever to roll the
armpits open, stretching the chest. Exhale, and lift one leg at a
time to the ceiling. Keep pulling the chair into the back as the
neck stretches. Eventually the body will be vertical; you will be
high on the shoulders. To release, place feet back to Plough
position. Move the chair at your back to one side, place your

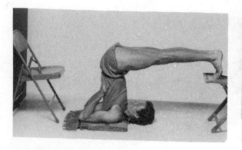
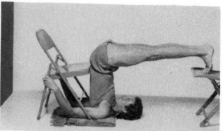
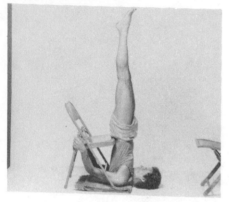

Clockwise From Top Left: Plough to Chair; Draw Chair Into Support Back; Lift Legs to Shoulder Stand

hands on the floor and roll the back down, one vertebra at a time. Keep the head on the floor. When legs are vertical, bend knees to chest, place feet on floor.

Benefits: Stretches chest, shoulders and neck. Aids student in learning correct Shoulder Stand and helps build time in inverted pose.

SPLIT LEG SHOULDER STAND

(Eka Pada Sarvangasana)

1. Placement. Begin in Shoulder Stand (see p. 156), hands on back.

2. Pose. Look at the right foot and visually gauge where it is in relation to the ceiling. Without moving the right leg in any way lower the left leg to the floor to the Plough position (see p. 158).

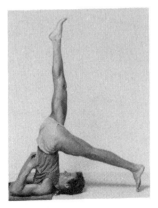 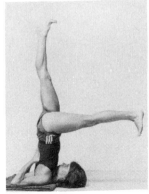 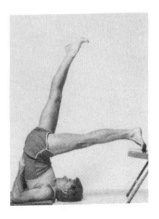

Split Leg Shoulder Stand-Pose   Horizontal Leg   Chair Support

Both knees are tight, the spine lifts toward ceiling. Do not allow the left hip to drop. Release any muscle contractions in the face, neck, and throat. Hold 5 to 10 seconds. Build to 30 seconds. Exhale, lift the leg. Reverse, hold for equal amount of time with each leg.

3. Variation. Do No. 2, but keep the left leg parallel to the floor (without taking the foot to the floor). Work on keeping the pelvic bones even. The thigh extends back, but not the hip.

4. Aid. Use a chair behind your head so that in No. 3 your foot will rest on chair.

Benefits: Strengthens and stretches legs and groins. Massages abdominal organs.

OPEN ANGLE SHOULDER STAND

1. Placement. Begin in Shoulder Stand (see p. 156), hands on back.

2. Pose. Exhale, open the legs to the sides. Keep feet squared, pull the kneecaps up toward groins. The entire spine lifts toward the ceiling as the legs lower.

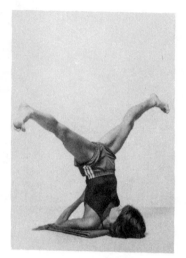

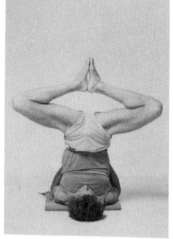

Open Angle Shoulder Stand-Pose   Soles of Feet Together

3. Variation. To rest the legs, bend the knees while bringing the soles of the feet together. The heels are as close to the groin as possible.

Benefits: Rests the legs while building time in Shoulder Stand. Stretches inner thigh muscles, develops balance.

EAR SQUEEZE

(Karnapidasana)

1. Placement. Do this pose only after you are quite comfortable in the Plough. Begin in the Plough, hands on rib cage.

2. Pose. Bend the knees and place them on the floor next to the ears. Turn the feet so the tops of the feet rest on the floor. With each exhalation relax more deeply into the pose. Hold 10 to 15 seconds, build to 1 minute.

3. Variation. For more stretch in the shoulders interlace fingers behind you. Stretch little fingers down to the floor and away from you.

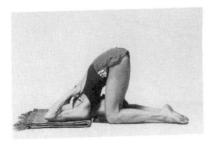 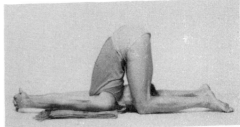

Ear Squeeze-Pose   Fingers Interlaced Stretching Away From Torso

4. Aid. If your hands don't touch behind you, hold a pole or cloth. As shoulders stretch, move hands toward each other.

Benefits: Stretches the back, rests the upper body and legs. Excellent resting pose during Shoulder Stand and Plough variations.

17

Humility: Sitting Forward Bends

The forward bending poses seem to capture the essential benefits of yoga: a strongly elongated body that houses a quiet mind. They are extremely beneficial for athletes because they give the entire back side of the body an intense stretch. These asanas (poses) teach tenacity, patience, and surrender, because these qualities are required for their successful execution. As the forward stretching is sustained, the complaining mind learns to surrender to the discomfort felt in the legs and in the back. This surrender can become a doorway to a quiet world within the body.

In the beginning, however, the yoga student does a forward bend and the legs immediately scream for a halt. This is the reaction of the powerful hamstring muscles. (Postures for elongating these muscles are given in "The Screamers: Hamstring Stretches" in Chapter 12.) The back is also given a terrific stretch by the forward bends. It is essential to protect the back by doing forward bends in the correct manner. The Stick Pose, (see p. 169) although not a forward bend, is included in this section to aid you in understanding the proper and safe way in which to bend.

Visualize the body in Stick Pose as a pocket knife with a blade opened to a 90 degree angle. The torso is the blade, the hips form the hinge, and the legs are the case. Allow the knife to close slowly. It bends at the hinges of the hips. The blade (torso) fits neatly just inside the case (legs). The trunk and legs are therefore

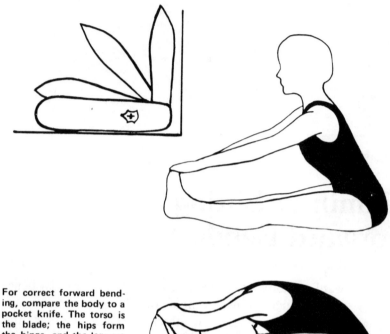

For correct forward bending, compare the body to a pocket knife. The torso is the blade; the hips form the hinge, and the legs are the case. Always bend from the hinge of the hips. The pelvis is in dog tilt.

in parallel planes. The arms come forward to hook the feet and to secure the position.

Let's examine the crucial factor in this closing movement—the efficiency of the bending point. In order for the body to stretch forward easily without damaging the back, several things must happen. The hamstrings, the calf muscles, and the muscles of the lower back must loosen. The pelvis must be tipped forward in a dog tilt. This pelvic tilt is most important. By sitting as far forward as possible on the sitting bones, and by continuing to push these bones away from the knees, the safety of the spine is guaranteed. The back will be flat like the straight edge of the knife's blade. If the forward bend is begun with the pelvis tilted back, as in the illustration, the legs are not stretched adequately, and the back receives a severe over-stretch. This incorrect movement makes practicing the pose dangerous instead of beneficial.

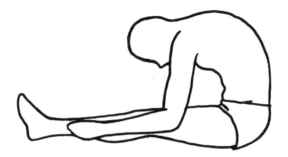

Incorrect forward bend-pelvis not in dog tilt, causing overstretch of the back.

As you do the Stick Pose and the forward bends, the feet must remain pushed equally away from you, they must be "squared" (see p. 29). The inner edge of the foot must receive exactly the same emphasis as the outer edge. Doing the Stick Pose with the feet against a wall will show you how to do this. *In all sitting forward bends keep the feet squared, even when holding the feet with the hands.*

Tenacity is required to hold these poses, and patience is developed and nurtured in that holding. As the forward bends are held for increasingly longer periods, the mind protests even more strongly against the discomfort. Eventually the mind learns to surrender to the poses. The surrender is developed only by many hours of practice, so do not be discouraged by the impatience that permeates your poses in the beginning.

Caution: When doing these poses do not attempt to close the torso to the legs in the beginning stages of your practice.

STICK POSE

(Dandasana)

1. Placement. Sit with the legs extended straight in line with your hips. *Feet, hips, shoulders in line and squared with a wall.*

2. Pose. Exhale, push feet away evenly, taking care to keep equal pressure on inner and outer feet. Press thighs to floor, legs remain straight, kneecaps pulled toward groin. Keep back erect by *sitting as far forward as possible on sitting bones, in dog tilt.* Palms flat on floor and in line with hips; fingers point to feet. Hold 15 to 20 seconds. Apply test for length in the back (see p. 122); no bones should be poking out at the back of the waist.

3. Aid. Sit on a pillow or rolled blanket, place a belt or tie around balls of feet. Hold ends of belt and use bent elbows and arms for leverage to keep spine erect. Pull the entire spine forward to vertical position.

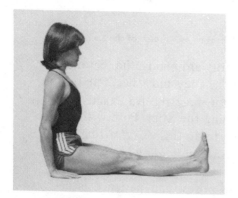

Stick Pose-Completed Pose;

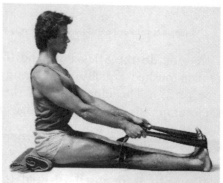

On Cushion With Belt

4. Aid. Do the Stick Pose with legs up the wall, buttocks touching or as close to wall as hamstrings will allow. Feet are turned as though standing on them, "squared" to ceiling. The pelvis is in gentle dog tilt. Flatten shoulder blades to floor, take sternum toward top of head, tuck chin slightly in, keeping face parallel to floor and ceiling. Palms flat on floor along body.

5. Aid. Sit on the floor opposite a folding chair. Place your feet against the back rung of the chair as pictured. Hold the seat of the chair with your hands and draw the entire torso forward, lifting the spine taller with each breath. Kneecaps must be tight. Heels and head lengthen away from buttocks.

Caution: Understanding and perfecting this pose is essential before proceeding to the forward bends.

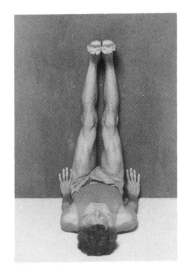

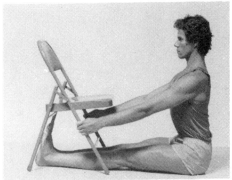

With Chair

Stick Pose Against Wall-Pose

If you cannot do Stick Pose with the vertebrae of the back forming an indented channel up the spine, then do all the following sitting poses with a roll under your buttocks. The roll should be high enough to tilt the pelvis *slightly* forward.

Benefits: Elongates and strengthens front and back of body equally. Stretches legs, strengthens back.

MOVING INTO THE STICK WITH THE WALL

1. Placement. Lie on your left side with the buttocks and feet touching the wall.

2. Pose. Exhale, roll on to your back, keeping the knees bent. Stretch the legs up the wall, keeping them straight. Come down by bending knees, feet flat on wall. Roll to left and sit up.

3. Variation. If this is impossible at first with straight legs, begin in No. 1 with buttocks about 1 or 2 feet from wall. This decreases stretch in hamstrings. Do No. 2.

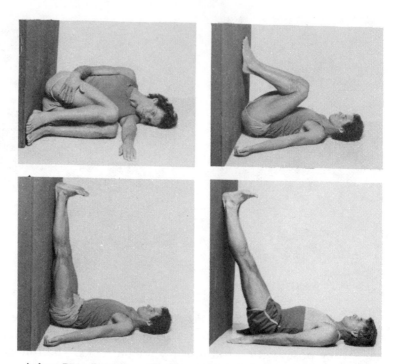

Left to Right From Top: Moving Into Stick Pose on Wall-Buttocks to Wall;
Roll to Back; Completed Pose; For Tight Hamstrings

HALF FORWARD BEND

(Janu Sirsasana)

1. Placement. Do the Stick Pose (see p. 169). Bend the right leg, bringing the heel to the buttock. Let the right leg drop to the side so it rests on its outer thigh and knee. Keep left leg extended and turned slightly in. Pelvic bones straight forward, spine erect.

2. Pose. Inhale, stretch up evenly with straight arms extended to ceiling. Feel the stretch originating from the hips. Exhale; *keeping pelvis in dog tilt, bend from the hips.* Sternum lies on knee with chin on shin. The vertical stretch of the torso has now become horizontal. Hold first the toes of extended foot, gradually extend your stretch to catch the sole, eventually holding wrists beyond

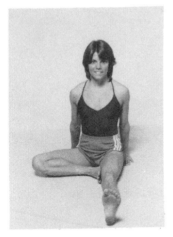
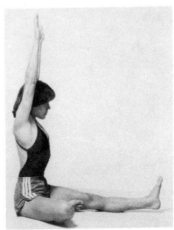

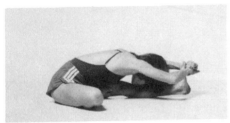

Clockwise From Top Left: Half Forward Bend-Placement; Arms and Torso
Extended Up; Completed Pose

foot. Trunk moves evenly along left leg (more stretching effort
must be made from the right hip to insure this equal movement).
Hold for a few breaths, release, and repeat for an equal amount of
time on the opposite side.

3. Variation. Do No. 2, but holding feet, on an inhalation
stretch the breastbone up, making the back concave. Do not take
body down again; simply work on achieving the concavity of the
back.

4. Aid. Place pillow under bent knee if it is not touching floor.
Using a belt around foot, hold both ends with hands and with elbows out pull the spine forward. Shoulders are low, away from
ears. Do No. 3.

Benefits: Gives intense stretch to extended leg. Opens hips.
Tones and stimulates internal organs. Strengthens and elongates
spine.

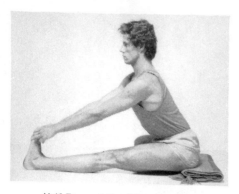

Half Forward Bend-Concave Back

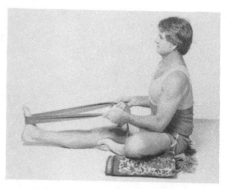

On Cushion with Belt

SEATED ANGLE POSE

(Upavistha Konasana)

1. Placement. Sit in the Stick Pose (see p. 169). Spread legs apart to a right angle, keeping them straight with heels pushed away evenly, feet squared. Kneecaps face ceiling. Stretch arms up, lift spine high.

2. Pose. Exhale, hold big toes with thumbs and next two fingers, keeping spine straight. Exhale, *in dog tilt, bend from hips, extending front and back of body evenly.* Head on floor. Eventually chest and chin on floor. Hold for a few breaths, working up to one minute. Up on inhalation.

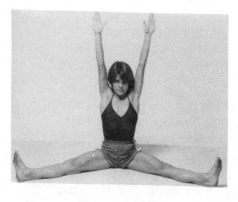

Seated Angle-Placement

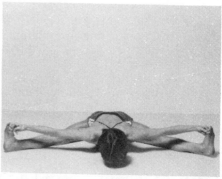

Completed Pose

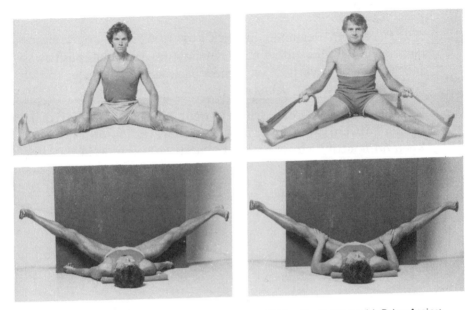

Left to Right From Top: Seated Angle Holding Thighs; On Cushion with Belts; Against Wall; Pressing Thighs

3. Variation. Do No. 1, hold inside thighs with fingers under thighs, elbows bent. Pull elbows back, using arms to lift and extend spine vertically. Torso is in Stick Pose. Shoulders moving down and back.

4. Aid. Wrap a belt around each foot, take the ends of the belt with each hand and in No. 3 continue pushing feet away while using belt to lift spine. Extend forward if possible. If the bones at the back of your waist stick out sit on rolled mat, do dog tilt. Another very useful way to practice this pose is with the legs on a wall. Begin as explained on p. 174, stretch legs up the wall in the Stick Pose, then widen the legs with feet "squared." Allow gravity to slowly loosen the inner thighs. To increase stretch place hands on inner thighs and gently press legs toward floor.

Caution: Consult a teacher if pain is felt in the inner knee during any variation of this pose.

Benefits: Stretches the legs, loosens the groins and hips. It is believed to offer special benefits to the female reproductive organs.

SIDE VARIATION OF OPEN ANGLE POSE

1. Placement. Beginning in Stick Pose (see p. 169), open legs to right angle. Do dog tilt so back remains straight. Heels push away and feet remain vertical or turned back slightly. Inhale, stretch both arms up by ears, palms in.

2. Pose Exhale, rotate trunk to right, keeping legs still. Exhale, stretch forward from hips, back flat, chin resting on right shin. Keep *both* sitting bones on floor. Hands hold foot as in Half Forward Bend (see p. 172). Hold for a few breaths, release and reverse.

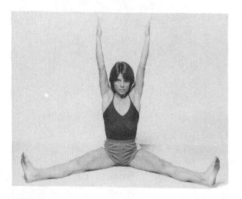
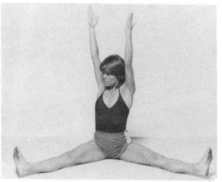
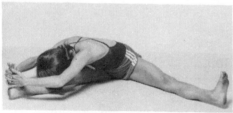

Clockwise From Top Left: Side Variation Open Angle Pose-Placement; Torso Rotated; Completed Pose

3. Variation. Do No. 1, rotate trunk to right. Hold right foot with both hands. Bend elbows, on inhalations open chest and elongate spine, on exhalations, take elbows out and move the elongated spine slightly downward. Work in this manner for several breaths. Do not disturb left foot. Release and reverse.

4. Aid. Sit on a rolled-up mat. Place belt around foot, use the belt to lengthen and stretch the trunk as in No. 3.

Benefits: Stretches inner thighs, groins, and hips. Both sides of torso given intense stretch.

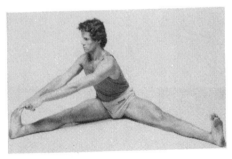

Side Variation Angle Pose-Extending Spine

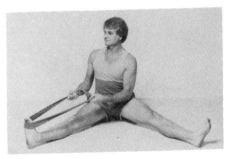

On Cushion with Belt

FULL FORWARD BEND

(Paschimottanasana)

1. Placement. Sit in the Stick Pose (see p. 169). Inhale, extend arms to ceiling, *pelvis in dog tilt.* Lift diaphragm.

2. Pose. Exhale, *bending at hips, maintain extended torso* and take hands to big toes. Ribs extend along legs toward top of head, face on shins. Gradually the extension will allow chin to rest on shins. Both sides of waist stretch evenly. Hold for a few breaths, working up to 1 minute. Inhale, come back to the Stick Pose, release.

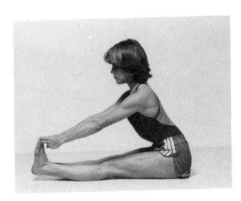

Full Forward Bend-Hand to Toes

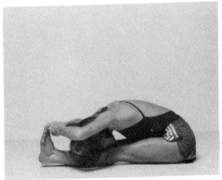

Extending to Completed Pose

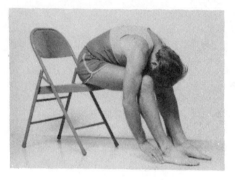

Full Forward Bend-Pose on Chair

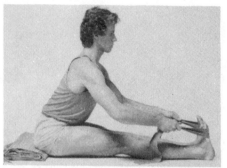

On Cushion with Belt Extending Back

3. Variation. Sit on edge of a hard chair, feet on floor in front of knees. (The more stretched your hamstrings are the straighter your legs can be.) Place feet parallel and wide as hips. Inhale, do No. 1. Exhale, bend from hips and extend breasts to knees, arms fall loosely to side. Remain in this position for as long as possible, allowing spine to lengthen and stretch.

4. Aid. Do the Stick Pose sitting on a pillow or rolled blanket. The pillow should be high enough to allow the bones at the back of your waist to be slightly indented while in Stick Pose. Place a belt or towel around the balls of the feet. On exhalations, continue moving elbows out and take breastbone toward toes, keeping back concave. Bend from hips. The spine moves forward.

Benefits: Intense stretch of entire backside of body. Massage given to abdominal organs. Calming effect when done correctly.

18

Revolve and Resolve: Twisting Poses

For many people, the word "yoga" instantly evokes images of pretzel bodies, knotted into impossible twists. Years of westernized abuse of yoga and a general misconception of the postures have led to this confusion.

Sometimes a student comes to yoga class with a desire to realize this contorted image with his or her own body. This student is inevitably disappointed to learn that the twisting poses are not designed to create human pretzels. Twists are not casually "slipped into"; neither should they be forced aggressively. They are done with the same precision and awareness that is demanded by all of the postures.

These *asanas* are not the exclusive domain of the experienced or more flexible student. These are twists that are possible and beneficial for the beginner. They can be especially useful in a yoga practice before or after competition because of their tension-relieving effects.

The essential principle of twisting postures is that *the spine must be elongated and not compressed as it turns.* So lift the spine toward the ceiling before turning. As you work with the twisting poses, remember that even though the spine is turning, it must also be extending. Visualize a spiral. Create space within the vertebrae as you twist.

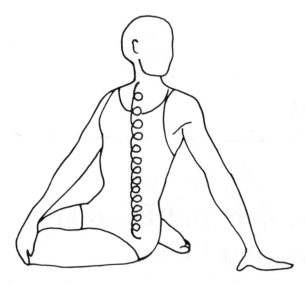

Twist by extending the spine, THEN turning. Visualize the spine making a spiral motion, one vertebra turning above the other.

Try this experiment. Stand with your feet about one foot apart and parallel. Without moving your feet, exhale, turning and twisting as far as you can to the left. Release to the center. Now before twisting to the right, first elongate the spine by tucking the tailbone down and lifting the sternum (breast bone), and extending both sides of the waist vertically. *Keep this extension, this upward movement* as you exhale, and turn to the right. Release to the center, continuing to move the spine upwards.

One way to check the extension of the spine is to keep the shoulders horizontal. Irregularities here indicate one side or the other of the spine is not stretching.

As you do twists, consider your spine as a spiral of gossamer thread that is growing longer and longer. Resist the sensation of a thick wire mattress coil that is compressed to support a 200 lb. weight! Also, never lead the twisting motion with the head. Simply allow the head to "follow" the direction of the twist. (If your head or neck hurts, you are pulling with head. Neck strain can result.)

Please note: People with medically proven herniated discs should not do twists.

CHAIR TWIST

1. Placement. Use a sturdy chair, preferably a folding type. Sit forward in the chair, feet parallel on the floor and slightly apart. The spine is straight, shoulders down and back, chin parallel to the floor.

2. Pose. Exhale, take the left hand behind you as far as possible on the back of the chair. Right hand holds back of chair. Both elbows are down. On exhalation, continue walking fingers to the left as you turn and *elongate the spine to the ceiling.* Keep the chest open and *do not move the feet.* Hold 15 seconds. Release slowly and reverse.

3. Variation. Sit on chair, facing left. Secure left knee against back of chair. Turn to left and hold chair back with both hands. Grow taller with each inhalation, turn to the left with each exhalation. Push with left hand, pull with right hand. Take left waist toward chair. With a little experimentation this twist can be done at the wheel of a car.

4. Aid. Use two thick books under your feet to enable you to keep the heels down.

Benefits: Teaches the twisting principle of extension during turning, releases tension in the spine.

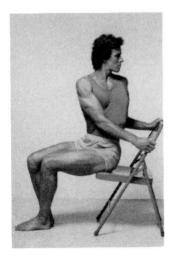 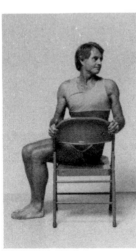 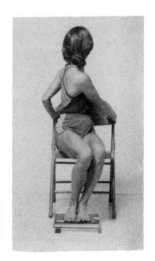

Chair Twist-Back to Chair   Side to Chair   Feet Supported

CROCODILE TWIST

1. Placement. Lie on your back, feet together, arms extended from shoulders, palms down. See that your body is straight and that you are forming a "t" position.

2. Pose. Exhale, push the heels away from you. Lift the right foot, wedging the right heel between the left big toe and second toe. Exhale; roll the feet to the left without disturbing the right foot's position. *Keep the shoulders flat and touching the floor.* Turn the head to the right. Allow the right hip to roll to the left, keep the left buttock in place. Soften the lower back. Hold for 10 to 15 seconds, release and reverse.

3. Variation. Place the arch of the right foot on top of the left knee. The left hand holds the right knee. Exhale; without disturbing the shoulders, take the right knee to the left. Head turns to right. Bring the breath high up in the chest to help lengthen the spine. Stretch the heel of the straight leg.

4. Aid. Place a sturdy piece of furniture near your hand and use this as an anchor for your arm and shoulder. Hold on to the furniture as you take the legs and hips in the opposite direction.

Benefits: Massages and revitalizes the spine, releases tension in the body.

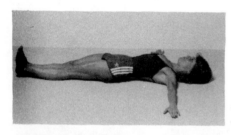
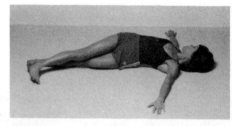
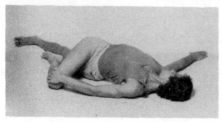
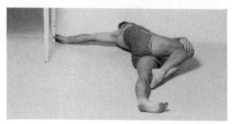

Left to Right from Top: Crocodile Twist-Placement; Heel on Toes; Arch to Knee; **Holding Anchor**

KNEE TO SIDE ROLLS

(preparation for Jathara Parivartanasana)

1. Placement. Lie on your back in Mountain Pose. Take your arms out to your side so that your body forms a "t." Arms form right angles with torso, palms down.

2. Pose. Exhale, bend both legs, knees to chest. Exhale, roll to right so that right knee touches floor. Take a few breaths and repeat to left. Come to center, release legs, then repeat cycle again.

3. Variation. Keep the feet flat on the floor near buttocks. Allow the feet to roll to the sides in order to take knees down.

4. Aid. Grip a sturdy piece of furniture with your left hand so that when you turn to the right, the left arm and shoulder will receive a stretch. Reverse the hold for the other side.

Benefits: Relieves back pain, tones abdominal area.

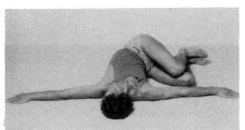 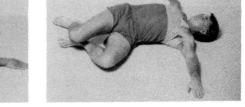

Knee to Side Rolls-Pose   Feet on Floor

BELLY TURNER

(Jathara Parivartanasana)

1. Placement. Lie on your back, arms extended with palms down, forming a "t" position. See that you are perfectly straight.

2. Pose. Exhale, bend both legs, bringing the knees to the chest. Exhale, take knees to the right side, then straighten legs on floor by pushing the heels away from you. Extend feet toward the right hand. *Keep left shoulder down, hips remain in line under*

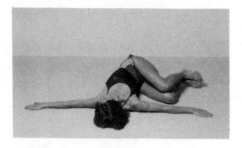

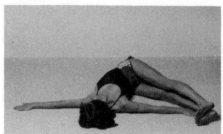

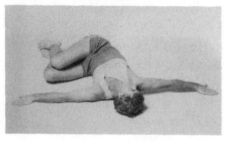

Clockwise From Top Left: Belly Turner-Knees to Side; Legs Straightened; Feet on Floor

shoulders. Move your navel to the left. Head turns to left. Hold 10 to 15 seconds. Exhale; bend the knees; come back to center and repeat on the left.

3. Variation. Do No. 2, bring knees to floor; do not straighten the legs.

Benefits: Strengthens and releases the back. Loosens hips. Massages the abdominal organs, firms the abdomen.

SIMPLE TWIST

(Bharadvajasana)

1. Placement. Sit on your heels, then shift the weight to the left and sit on the left buttock. Keeping the left leg under the right thigh, place the right hand on the left knee. Place the left hand to the left in line with the left thigh, fingers pointing backwards.

2. Pose. Exhale; press down with the hands and turn the entire body to the left, rolling the right hip forward. Extend the sternum up, keeping the shoulders down and back. *Keep the spine straight;*

}

do not lean to the left. Walk the left fingers around towards right hip to help you twist. Retaining the twist, take the right buttock back to the floor. Hold for 10 to 15 seconds. Release slowly and reverse.

3. Variation. Do No. 2, but keep the right hip rolled forward, the right buttock remaining off the floor.

4. Aid. Sit six inches away from wall in position No. 1, left thigh beside wall. Turn left to face wall, placing your hands on the wall at shoulder level. Use your hands to aid your twist, keeping the spine straight and parallel with the wall. Vary this by beginning with the left thigh touching the wall, turning the chest to touch the wall, shoulders square to the wall.

Benefits: Increases the flexibility of the entire spine.

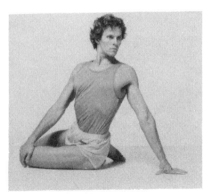
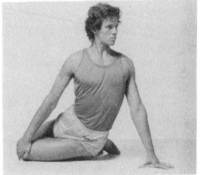
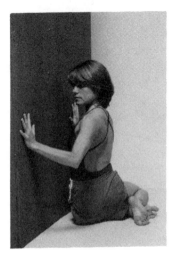

Clockwise From Top Left: Simple Twist-Pose with Hips Down; With Hip Rolled Forward; With Wall as Lever

TWIST

(Marichyasana I)

1. Placement. Sit in Stick pose (see p. 169). Exhale, bring left heel to right groin. Left shin is perpendicular to floor.

2. Pose. Inhale, stretch spine upward, concaving back. Inhale, take left arm straight up, then exhale, stretch left arm over left knee. Left armpit extends over knee, moving toward left shin with no space between the left side of the body and the left knee. Throw the left forearm back along the waist. Extend the right hand to clasp either the fingers, hands or wrists. Turn to the right. Open chest, concave back. Keep left buttock on floor. Throat and eyes remain loose. Hold 10 to 20 seconds. Return to center, release and reverse for same length of time.

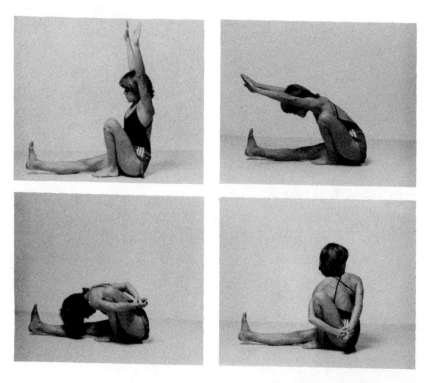

Left to Right From Top: Twist-Stretch Arms and Spine UP; Extend Forward; Left Hand Holds Right Wrist; Sit Tall and Twist

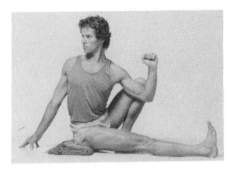

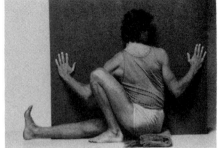

Twist on Mat, Arms Working   Against Wall

3. Variation. Sit on a rolled up mat. Do No. 2, but do not hold hands. Keep the right fingers on the floor as in the Simple Twist, (see p. 184). Bend the left elbow, forearm perpendicular to floor, make a fist and pressing the elbow into the knee turn the torso.

4. Aid. Do No. 2 with right leg and buttock touching wall. Keep both arms bent with hands on wall. Use the hands and arms to get the shoulders squared with the wall.

Benefits: Tones and massages abdominal area. Relieves back pain.

19

Wake Up: Sun Salutation

The Sun Salutation is a combination of poses done by moving smoothly from one to the other while coordinating the breath. There are many combinations possible; the version given here is a more traditional one.

Before doing the Sun Salute be sure to practice each of these poses as they were presented earlier. Once you have some understanding of each individual pose in the series you may wish to use the Sun Salute as a morning warm-up, as it is traditionally intended, or as a general warm-up before any athletic activity.

By looking at the poses you will see why the Sun Salute is an excellent warm-up for the total body. The series begins in the Mountain Pose, so alignment is established. This is followed by forward bending, backbending and groin stretches. The arms and wrists are strengthened and stretched in the Squeeze, "Push-Down," Dog Pose. The back is lengthened, the chest opened. Awareness is directed to the breath. Practicing the series until it flows smoothly increases flexibility, strength, and coordination.

In some cases the photos show two "versions" of each individual pose. One photo indicates how a stronger, more flexible individual can do the Sun Salute. The other photos show a less rigorous variation. Everyone should do the easier version first, and then work into the harder version as you are more able to do so. The backbending poses are the ones you should be most careful with. If you don't have a teacher and you have a weak back *only do the easier version for 3 or 4 months.*

Because the legs are stepped back one at a time you must always balance the body by doing this Sun Salute at least twice, the first time stepping back with one leg, the second time stepping with the other leg. Also, although this is meant to be done by moving from one pose to the next with each breath, you may do the Sun Salute more slowly by holding each posture. Use the breath to get into the pose and then breathe evenly as you hold. It should help you to remember when to inhale and when to exhale if you know, in general, to inhale on back bending poses and exhale on forward bending poses.

These poses have been explained before so there is a page reference for the previous instructions. Emphasis here will be on the breath, the guiding force from one pose to the next.

SUN SALUTATION

(Suryanamasgar)

1. Mountain Pose. Align and breathe evenly.

2. Inhale, turn palms out, stretch fingers down and spine up.

3. Indian Greeting (Namaste). Exhale, place palms together, straight line from elbow to elbow. Shoulders wide.

4. Inhale, stretch arms overhead, eyes gaze at hands. To arch the back be sure buttocks are squeezed firmly in cat tilt, then the upper spine moves forward as the chest stretches open. Note that in the easier variation the head is turned only slightly up and the shoulders are low. The pelvis is tucked in cat tilt but do not arch the back.

5. Standing Forward Bend (see p. 140). Exhale slowly as you bend forward, arms in line with torso.

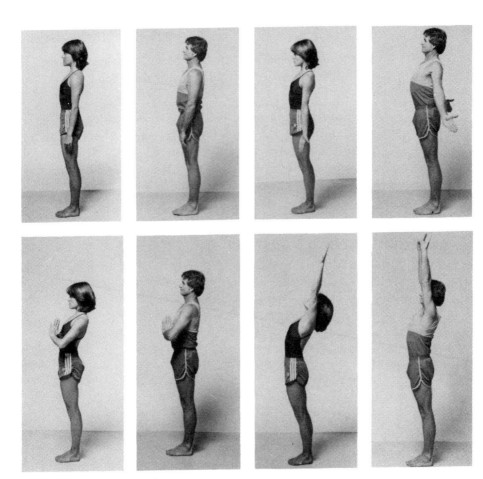

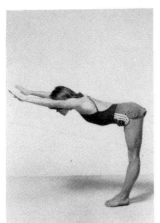

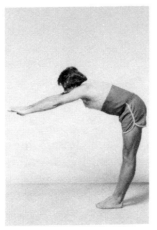

Left to Right From Top:
Sun Salutation; Mountain
Pose; Palms Turn Out;
Palm To Palm; Stretch
Arms Up; Bending For-
ward

6. Hands are placed next to the feet, arms are straight. If your legs are tight hang down for a moment then bend your knees so hands reach the floor.

7. Forward Lunge (see p. 102). Inhale. Bend the left knee to a right angle and step the right foot back, turn the toes under. Bring the buttocks down so body is straight from head to heel. Lengthen spine, do not collapse chest. Alternate version: back leg may bend slightly, or even the knee may rest on the floor.

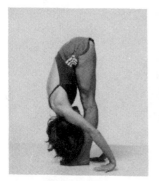
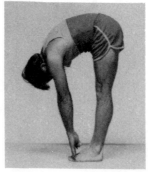
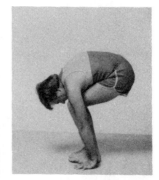
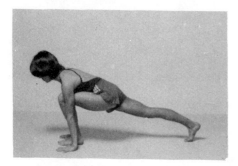
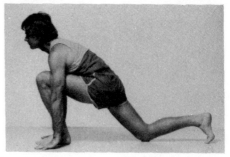

Left to Right From Top: Standing Intense Stretch of Back; Bend Knees to Place Hands on Floor; Forward Lunge; Lunge with Knee Bent

8. Push-Up Position. Retain the breath, step the other foot back. Pelvis is in cat tilt. Hands point directly forward. Shoulder blades are flat. Shoulders are away from ears.

9. Squeeze Position. The spine recoils now. Exhale, bend the elbows and knees, tip the buttocks up in dog tilt, and lower yourself to the floor so the knees, chest, and chin touch simultaneously. The easier version uses the "Bent Knee Push-Up" position

(see p. 71). The pelvis is tucked in cat tilt. Lower with control then lie on floor, straighten legs.

10. Upward Dog (see p. 149). Inhale, straighten the arms and lengthen the spine in Upward Dog. The pelvis is firmly tucked in cat tilt, the entire torso is off the floor. Look only slightly up. The alternate version uses Preparation for Cobra (see p. 145). Again, do not compress the neck by looking up; look forward or slightly down so back of neck is long.

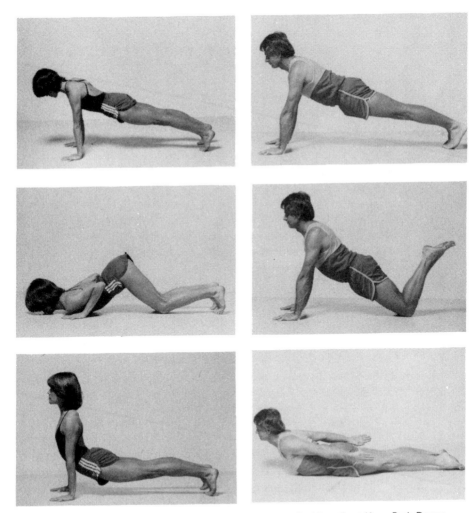

Left to Right From Top: Push Up Position; Squeeze Position; Bent Knee Push-Down; Upward Dog; Preparation for Cobra

11. Downward Dog (see p. 125). Exhale, lift the buttocks in dog tilt, lower armpits toward floor. Press on the heel of the hands, lengthen the spine. When doing the easier version do the "Bent Knee Push-Up" (see p. 71), then place toes on floor, straighten legs and lift buttocks to Downward Dog position. Stay high up on toes.

12. Forward Lunge (see p. 102). Inhale, bend the right knee and step the right foot forward, placing the foot between the hands. Buttocks are in cat tilt so body is in a straight line. Alternate version: Back leg may be bent slightly.

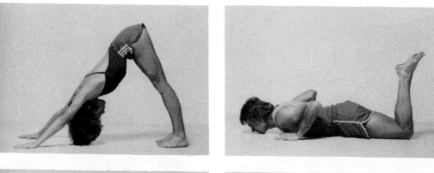

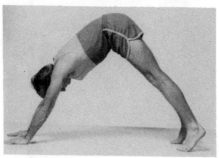
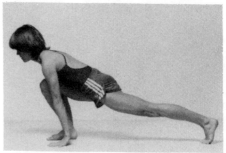

Left to Right From Top: Downward Dog; Bent Knee Push-Up; Downward Dog-Heels Up; Forward Lunge

13. Standing Forward Bend (see p. 140). Exhale, straighten the right leg and bring the left foot next to the right. Lift the buttocks high in dog tilt, kneecaps are tight. In the alternate version, let the hands leave the floor but keep lifting the buttock bones with knees tight. If hamstrings are very tight, bend the knees slightly.

14. Mountain Pose, arms overhead. Inhale, with the arms overhead lift the spine as a single unit and stand. The alternate way to

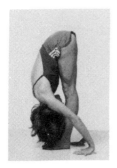
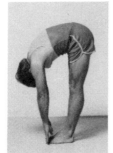
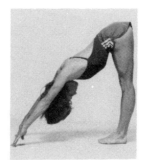
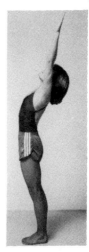

Left to Right: Standing Forward Bend; Same Pose Done by Beginner; Preparation to Stand; Mountain Pose With Arms Up.

stand is to leave the arms hanging, tuck the pelvis down in cat tilt, and roll the spine up one vertebra at a time. Head lifts last.

15. Indian Greeting (Namaste). Exhale, bend the elbows and place hands palm to palm in front of chest.

16. Mountain Pose. Lower arms to sides. Realign and breathe evenly.

Benefits: Excellent overall warm-up that brings flexibility to the spine and legs, stretches the chest, strengthens the arms and shoulders. Develops coordination and breath control.

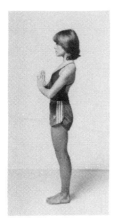
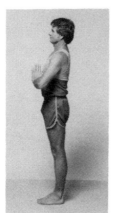
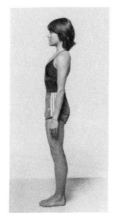
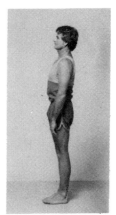

Palm to Palm   Mountain Pose

20

Resting Poses

For physical, mental, and emotional balance you usually need to rest after each and every yoga practice and/or workout. With the exception of the nerve cells the entire body is constantly being regenerated; old cells die and slough off, new cells replace them. The nerve cells, however, are with us from cradle to grave. Because of its longevity the nervous system needs rest. A yoga relaxation uses the mind to turn off muscle after muscle, thereby minimizing the bombardment of nervous impulses being conducted by the system. Once you have acquired the knack of it, a ten minute relaxation can leave you more refreshed than an hour's nap.

Physiologically, resting after a calisthenic-type workout is essential to eliminate fatigue. As muscles contract no oxygen is consumed, nor carbon dioxide produced, and the lactic acid content increases. Upon relaxing the muscle and bringing oxygen to it via the respiratory system the lactic acid content decreases. In most physical activities the respiratory system can't supply adequate oxygen to fully eliminate lactic acid, and so fatigue results. Resting for even a minimal amount of time will reduce these effects. This may make an enormous difference in your attitude toward your workout.

Psychologically you need to relax. Tension literally lives in your body. It is reflected in a tight belly, clenched jaw, furrowed brow; abundant unnecessary muscle contractions that sap your energy and wear away at your nervous systems. But what to do? How do you begin to let go, to free yourself of what seems to be self-perpetuating tension? By relaxation! With practice it can be learned.

First, do some yoga poses to release muscular tension. The harder you work, the more complete the relaxation. Then assume a comfortable position (see Corpse Pose p. 200) in a quiet spot. You must then feel inwardly for any areas you are contracting. To attain relaxation the mind must first "see" the tension and then allow for its softening.

Relaxation is not something we can feign nor is it something we can force; it has to be genuine and pursued patiently or it eludes us. This is why relaxation is the ultimate tool in blending the body and mind, because relaxation is like quicksilver. With only the slightest wavering, only a moment's wandering of the mind the muscles can contract and draw us into a nervous state again. To relax, both the body and the brain must cooperate, must be one with the other, yoked. When this happens we become whole.

Frequent experiences of relaxation begin to generalize to all else that we do. Even in conducting the business of living, there is a calmness that underlies all action. Just as tension lives in our bodies so does calmness. It is manifest by contracting only the muscles necessary for movement, by an even breath, by a mind capable of concentration and creativity, by a loving spirit. In athletics we call this efficiency, in medicine we call this health, in living we call this comfort.

So relaxation has lots to offer if only you will take the time to do it—classic directions say at least ten to twenty minutes. How about one to two minutes at first? When doing the Corpse Pose begin by just focusing on your breath. Watch it, don't change it. Feel your body grow heavier; gravity is real; it is drawing every cell in your body toward the center of the earth. Feel yourself loosen as you let go. Then begin at your toes and work methodically up your body feeling the toes, the soles, and so on up to the crown of the head. There's nothing magical about relaxation; with time and proper attention, it's yours.

CHILD'S POSE

(Darnikasana)

1. *Placement.* Sit on mat in Preparation for Hero's Pose (see p. 81), knees together, feet parallel and apart slightly. Lengthen spine, without over-arching do dog tilt with pelvis.

2. *Pose.* Bend at the groin and stretch the torso forward until the forehead rests on the mat. Tuck chin in slightly to lengthen neck. Place hands by feet, palms up. Relax face, neck, shoulders, arms, hands, stomach. Feel gravity draw you toward the earth.

3. *Aid.* If legs are tight and prevent relaxing, place a cushion between the feet and buttocks. Do not let the cushion be so large that the body weight goes too far forward onto the forehead. The weight should be distributed evenly from head to toes. If the head does not touch the floor put cushion under head.

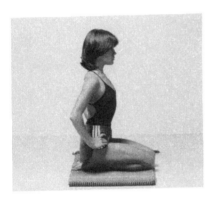
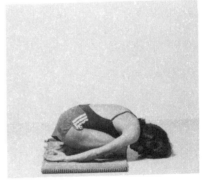
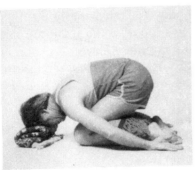

Clockwise From Top Left: Child's Pose-Placement; Completed Pose; Pad Into Knees, Head Supported

4. Aid. If you are tight in the groin place a rolled towel across both groins. Pull back on the towel as you bend the torso over it. Most pain is caused by compression; this aid may help to make space and relieve the pressure.

Benefits: Releases tension in lower back. Useful particularly after sitting forward bends and back bending.

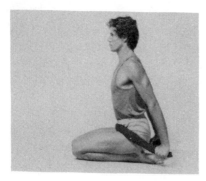

Child's pose-Towel Across Groin

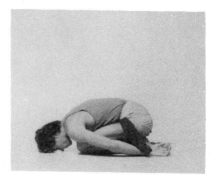

Pose

CORPSE POSE

(Savasana)

1. Placement. Lie on your back in a straight line. Tuck the pelvis down in cat tilt. The feet are about 18 inches apart, toes falling out. Hands are about a foot away from thighs, palms up. The eyes are closed.

2. Pose. Be perfectly still and feel inwardly. Breathe, relaxing with each exhalation. Let the entire body and particularly the eyes sink back toward the earth. The jaw is loose so the teeth are not touching; the tongue is broad in the mouth. Release any and all voluntary contractions. As the body softens it will lengthen. Note how the mind wanders, then refocus on the body. Hold 5 to 20 minutes.

3. Aid. If your chin is higher than your forehead in this pose, place a slim book, folded towel or cushion under the back of the head. The face should be parallel to the floor.

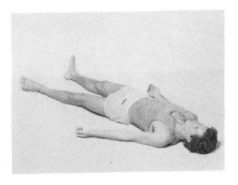

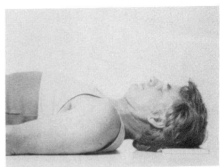

Corpse Pose-Completed Pose;   Book Under Head to Lower Chin

4. Aid. Lying on the back causes the lower back to arch slightly. If your back aches for any reason, place the lower legs on a chair. Or, if necessary, simply bend the knees and place both feet on the floor. Lifting or bending the legs this way flattens the back and usually will relieve any discomfort.

5. Aid. To enhance breathing and open the chest use a rolled up towel under the back bone. The towel should be placed at the lower back, extend up the spine and support the head.

6. Aid. Ideally this should be done in the dark so the eyes can fully relax. Put a folded towel across your eyes if you're in the direct sunlight or under bright lights.

Benefits: Relaxes and refreshes all systems of the body. Blends body and mind, brings awareness of mental and physical tension.

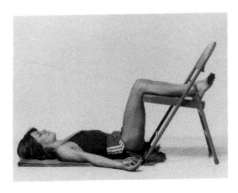

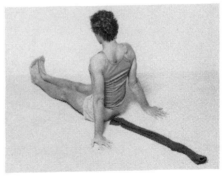

Lowers Legs on Chair for Complaining Back;   Towel Under Spine for Chest Expansion

Appendix

Practice Guide

There are ten stages in this guide. Progression from one stage to the next should be determined by how you *feel*. If you have changed some, if you have gained some flexibility and have some understanding of the poses in each stage, then continue to the next. How fast you progress depends on so many things: how much time you spend practicing, correct practice, how flexible and strong you are at the beginning, what you've done in the past (the body has a way of remembering), your emotional state, other physical activities you are doing. In general, if you are doing yoga regularly, as often as you work out or four times a week, work on each stage for three or four weeks. The first stage requires less time.

You can always go backward in the sequence but never jump forward skipping one or more stages. Judge your readiness for the next stage not only on flexibility but also on strength. If you are doing *yoga*, not just grinding out stretches, you will never be bored, but if you find you are complacent, move on. If you decide to do your own routine begin with at least three or more of the standing poses and then follow the sequence of the poses as they are arranged within each section, and by section. Above all, *never do a Shoulder Stand without being thoroughly warmed up.*

End all practice sessions with at least five minutes of the Corpse Pose.

Stage I.

  Pelvic Tilting
  Knee Lifts
  Squaring the feet
  Mountain Pose
  Tree Pose
  Jumping
  Standing Side Stretch
  Triangle Pose
  Hamstring Flexibility Test
  Neck Stretch
  Stick Pose with feet up the wall
  Chest Opener
  Full Body Stretch
  Corpse Pose

Stage II. Add to the above:

  Warrior II
  Beginning Leg Lifts
  Hamstring Stretch, Beginners and Knee to Chest
  Sink Stretch for Back, probably on knees
  Wrist Stretch
  Tailor Pose
  Prone Back Stretch
  Locust
  Preparation for Cobra
  Child's Pose
  Hare Pose
  Bound Angle up wall
  Shoulder Stand with wall, keep feet on wall
  Knees to Chest
  Crocodile Twist

Stage III. Add to the above:

  Extended Lateral Pose
  Spread Leg Forward Bend with chair
  Achilles, Calf Stretch
  Sink Stretch for Groin
  Hand Clasp
  Arm Stretch standing
  Progressive Hamstring Stretch

Sink Stretch for Achilles and Calves
Feet Stretches
    Fingers and Toes Entwined
    Foot Extensions
    Preparation for Hero's Pose
Bound Angle
Sit Ups

Stage IV. Consolidate, work on hardest poses. Add:
Push-Up appropriate to your strength
Lunge Groin Stretch
Spinal Roll
Full Sitting Forward Bend on chair

Stage V. Add:
Intense Side Stretch
Scissor Stretch
Sitting Leg Stretch
Squat Series
Lunge Groin Stretch
Supported Back Stretch
Shoulder Stand, one foot off the wall at a time
Stick Pose
Chair Twist

Stage VI. Add:
Wall Hang
Hand to Foot with towel
Runner's Warm Up
Cow's Head — arms only
Thigh Strengthener
Door Stretch for back
The Bridge
Crossed Leg Spinal Roll
Open Angle Pose up the wall
Shoulder Stand both feet off wall
Knee to Side Rolls
Simple Twist

Stage VII. Add:
Warrior I
Revolved Triangle
Reclined Side Stretch

The Gate Pose
Hand to Foot
Downward Dog with chair
The Camel
Table Pull ups
Hero's Pose
Shoulder Stand without wall
Stomach Turner

Stage VIII. Add:

Half Moon
Standing Intense Stretch for Back
Reclining Hero
Downward Dog on Floor
Upward Facing Dog
Boat Pose
Shoulder Stand with chairs
Plough with wall
Half Sitting Forward Bend
Intense Front Stretch
Full Body Sitting Forward Bend

Stage IX. Add:

Warrior III
Extended Toe to Hand Pose
Sitting on Nothing at All
Butterfly Stretch
Leg Lifts
Preparation for Half Lotus
Hero's Pose Groin and Knee Stretch
Open Angle Pose
Split Leg Shoulder Stand
Supine Hand to Foot (Supta Pagangusthasana)
Twist

Stage X. Add:

Sun Salute
Sitting Bow Pose
Standing Half Bow
Bow Pose
Open Angle Shoulder Stand
Ear Squeeze
Side Variation Open Angle

Core Program

Here are basic poses to keep a minimal amount of stretch in the major muscles and joints of the body. Because easier variations have been presented for each of these poses you can use this program no matter how flexible you may be. Be sure to add to this list those poses you have found that are essential to keep your "tight spots" pliable. This list is purposely short so that it is practical for you to do regularly.

Mountain Pose (Tadasana)
Triangle Pose (Trikonasana)
Extended Lateral Pose (Parsvokonasana)
Standing Intense Stretch of Back (Uttanasana)
Downward Dog (Adho Mukha Svanasana)
Upward Dog (Urdhva Mukha Svanasana)
Squat Series
Leg Lifts (Urdhva Prasarita Padasana)
Shoulder Stand (Sarvangasana)
Plough (Halasana)
Knees to Chest (Apanasana)
Progressive Hamstring Stretch or Supine Hand to Foot
    (Supta Padandusthasana)
Bound Angle (Badha Konasana)
Full Forward Bend (Paschimottanasana)
Crocodile Twist
Corpse Pose (Savasana)

Suggested Routine Before and After Running

Mountain Pose
Triangle Pose
Extended Lateral Pose
Downward Dog: Variation appropriate to you
Squat Series
Hero's Pose: Variation appropriate to you
Runner's Warm-Up
Walk
Run
Walk
Pelvic Tilting
Wall Hang
Spread Foot Forward Bend
Downward Dog
Sink Stretch for Back with or without partner
Sink Stretch for Achilles
Sink Stretch for Groin
Hero's Pose
Bound Angle with wall
Open Angle with wall
Shoulder Stand with or without wall
Plough with or without wall
Crocodile Twist
Corpse Pose

Areas of Concentration for Various Sports

These poses are chosen to add strength and stretch where you need it for your sport and to compensate for imbalances. By adding these poses to the Core Program (see p. 209) yoga will increase your athletic performance, enhance overall health and decrease the chance of injury.

Walking and running

For flexibility: preliminary hamstring stretches, standing poses, all forward bends, feet stretches, hip and groin stretches, backbends.

For strength: standing poses, thigh strengthener, Downward Dog, push-ups, table pull-ups, leg lifts, sit ups.

Bicycling

For flexibility: standing poses, preliminary hamstring stretches, all forward bending poses, chest opener, Hero's Pose and its variations, all groin stretches especially Standing Half Bow, back stretches, backbending, Shoulder Stand important to stretch back of neck.

For strength: push-ups, table pull-ups, preparation for Cobra, Locust, Shoulder Stand.

Horseback Riding

For flexibility: pelvic tilting, standing poses, preliminary hamstring stretches, Bound Angle, Open Angle, all groin stretches, feet stretches and particularly Hero's Pose and its variations, back stretches, twists.

For strength: standing poses, push-ups, pull-ups, stomach strengtheners, Locust, preparation for Cobra, Shoulder Stand.

Ballet and Modern Dancing

For flexibility: pelvic tilting, Achilles Sink Stretch, Achilles-Calf Stretch, squat series, forward bending poses with attention to alignment of the feet, Hero's Pose, back stretches.

For strength: standing poses, push-ups, pull-ups, inverted poses.

Folk and Square Dancing

For flexibility: pelvic tilting, standing poses, preliminary hamstring stretches, all poses for feet, knees and lower legs, all forward bending poses, back stretches.

For strength: standing poses, push-ups, pull-ups, stomach strengtheners, Shoulder Stand.

Gymnastics

For flexibility: all the stretching poses will enhance your flexibility.

For strength: standing poses, pelvic tilting, all stomach strengtheners are very important.

Water Skiing

For flexibility: standing poses, stretches for shoulders and arms, poses for feet, knees, and lower legs, all forward bending poses, back stretches, backbending twists.

For strength: stomach strengtheners.

Weight Lifting

For flexibility: all stretches in this book; pay particular attention to pelvic tilting, spinal alignment, feet stretches. Do all back stretches religiously!!!

Racquet Sports

These are difficult to balance because they are so one-sided. For true balance it would be necessary to play equal amounts of time using the non-dominant arm. So stretch your dominant side more and strengthen the non-dominant side as much as possible.

For flexibility: standing poses, all forward bending poses, particularly Spread Leg Forward Bend with arms overhead, all shoulder and arm stretches, Wrist Stretch, Squat Series, Hero's Pose and all its variations, stretches for lower legs, hips and thighs, back stretches, backbending. To help prevent tennis elbow do Plough Pose, variation 4 or 5 frequently!!!

For strength: standing poses, Thigh Strengthener, sit-ups, pull-ups.

Soccer

For flexibility: same as for runners and particularly Hero's Pose and its variations, groin stretches, Downward Dog and all back stretches. Do Shoulder Stand and Plough to stretch neck after heading.

For strength: Thigh Strengthener, standing poses, stomach strengtheners, pull-ups.

Ice Skating

For flexibility: back stretches, all poses for feet, knees, lower legs, all forward bending poses.

For strength: stomach strengtheners, pull-ups, Downward Dog, Shoulder Stand.

Swimming

For flexibility: Achilles and Calf Stretch, Squat Series Hero's Pose and all its variations especially good for ankles and feet, all forward bending poses, all backbending poses, twists, stretches for shoulders and arms.

For strength: standing poses, inverted poses, stomach strengtheners.

Boating

For flexibility: hand clasp, wrist stretch, back stretches, all forward bending poses, all backbending poses, twists, groin stretches.

For strength: standing poses, preparation for Cobra, Locust.

Bowling

For flexibility: Poses from each section of this book. Chest Opener, back stretches, shoulder and arm stretches, twists.

For strength: stomach strengtheners, standing poses, pull-ups, push-ups.

Backpacking

For flexibility: preliminary hamstring stretches, all forward bending poses, back stretches, all feet and ankle poses, all shoulder and arm poses, backbending poses.

For strength: standing poses, Thigh Strengthener, stomach strengthener, pull-ups.

Golf

Because of twisting while swinging, low back pain is a common complaint. To remedy, pay careful attention to alignment in all poses and learn to twist correctly; read the introduction to the twisting section carefully.

For flexibility: pelvic tilting, Hand Clasp, Wrist Stretch, back stretches, all hamstring stretches, backbending poses, all twisting poses.

For strength: standing poses, belly strengtheners, Thigh Strengthener, Preparation for Cobra, Locust.

Downhill Skiing

For flexibility: standing poses especially Triangle, Warrior I,

Warrior II; groin stretches, hamstring stretches, back stretches, backbends, twists.

For strength: stomach strengtheners, arm strengtheners, Preparation for Cobra, Locust.

Cross-Country Skiing

For flexibility: pelvic tilting, Hero's Pose and its variations, groin stretches, forward and backbending poses, all hamstring stretches, squat series, back stretches, Chest Opener, Cow Pose.

For strength: standing poses, Preparation for Cobra, Locust.

Basketball

Do all the same poses as recommended for runners. Strong emphasis on standing poses with careful attention to knees. Do lots of back stretches and long Shoulder Stands. *Build* time in Thigh Strengthener.

Softball

Do poses from each section of this book. Stretches for arms especially, Spread Leg Forward Bend with arms overhead, Cow's Face, Plough with hands to floor, Wrist Stretch.

Volleyball

Do poses from each section of this book. Back stretches are important.

Cervical (7)
(Neck-Concave Curve)

Thoracic (12)
(Ribcage-Convex Curve)

Lumbar (5)
(Waist-Concave Curve)

Sacral-Coccygeal (9)
(Tailbone-Convex Curve)

Lateral View-Four curves of the vertebral column

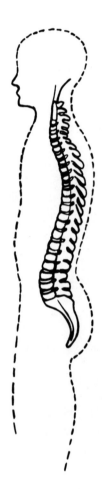

Glossary

Asana — Pose, posture held comfortably.

Balance — Skeletal-muscular equilibrium which facilitates maximum strength and flexibility; results in mental awareness of body.

Cat tilt — Position of pelvis where tailbone is tucked down.

Dog tilt — Position of pelvis where tailbone is lifted away from knees.

Hatha yoga — Use of physical poses to unify body, mind, spirit.

Lengthen — Stretch, make space in the body.

Namaste — Indian greeting with hands palm to palm. Means "I salute your soul."

Open — Stretch, make space. For example, open the chest by lifting breast bone, moving shoulders back and down, lifting rib cage off of pelvis.

Pranayama — Rhythmic control of breath.

S curve — Natural shape of back; rib cage area and tail bone are convex curves, neck and waist area are concave curves.

Sitting bones — The two single bones at the bottom of each buttock, where you sit. Particularly important because the hamstrings attach to these bones. The anatomical name for them is ischial tuberosity.

Stretch reflex — Shortening reaction of any muscle that is stretched too fast or too far.

Tadasana — Basic standing pose that teaches correct alignment of feet, legs, entire spine, head.

Bibliography

Light on Yoga by B.K.S. Iyengar. Schocken Books, New York, 1966. (Revised edition, 1977.) The yogic approach to total health is clearly outlined by Mr. Iyengar, a teacher with over forty years of experience. Over 600 illustrations accompany his detailed *asana* (pose) and *pranayama* (breathing) instructions. A succinct yoga philosophy chapter introduces the postures, followed by a self-study course outline. Specific postures are suggested for relieving various health problems. A dependable guide for the beginner, a definitive reference for the serious practitioner.

Inner Beauty, Inner Light by Frederick Leboyer. Alfred A. Knopf, New York, 1978. An exquisite gem that reflects the many facets of yoga. Leboyer has written a book on yoga for pregnant women, but any yoga student will appreciate his accurate photography and his imaginative prose. B.K.S. Iyengar has written the foreword, and Iyengar's daughter, Vanita, demonstrates the asanas during the last weeks of her pregnancy. Iyengar's precise and demanding approach to yoga is seen throughout the book.

Structural Yoga by Mukunda (Tom Stiles). Collected Consciousness, Davis, Calif., 1976. Excellent text on how to analyze your own structure and specific guide for poses to remedy imbalances. Particularly useful if you don't have a teacher.

Hatha Yoga for Complete Health by Sue Luby. Prentice-Hall, New Jersey, 1977. A book that has useful anatomical drawings of correct and incorrect movement. Photographs with arrowed movement lines illustrate the different stages of entering pose and how energy moves in poses.

Yoga Journal, 2054 University Ave., Berkeley, Calif. 94704. A bimontly publication of the California Yoga Teachers Association. A magazine that represents a broad range of yoga interests and tastes. Regular features include "Commentaries on Teaching," "Readers Forum," and a very useful practice guide that features an individual asana (pose) in each issue.

Yoga for People Over 50 by Suza Norton. Devin-Adair Co., Old Greenwich, 1977. Not just for the over-50 age group. This book expresses excellent thoughts on yoga philosophy and gives practical advice for doing the asanas. A gentle yoga book that incorporates Iyengar-style alignment.

New Exercises for Runners from the editors of *Runner's World.* World Publications, Mountain View, Calif., 1978. More pictures and explanations of Iyengar yoga poses, particularly clear guide to standing poses.

Yoga and the Athlete by Ian Jackson. World Publications, Mountain View, Calif., 1975. Personal story of how an avid runner turned to yoga to prevent continual injuries. Relates interesting accounts of working with yoga teachers—Felicity Hall, J.B. Rishi, B.K.S. Iyengar, Joel Kramer.

Stretching by Bob Anderson. Published by the author, Fullerton, Calif., 1975. Numerous stretches with routines for specific athletes.

Low Back Pain Syndrome by Rene Caillet. F.A. Davis Co., 1962. Medicines' view of the back. Highly anatomical but essential information on back care.

Rolfing by Ida Rolf. Dennis-Landman, Santa Monica, Calif., 1977. An excellent description of what the healthy body should be like. Pictures of people in and out of alignment and explanations of the causes.

The Foot Book by Harry F. Hlavac. World Publications, Mountain

View, Calif., 1977. Thorough, technical explanation of feet, imbalances and what to do about them.

Touch for Health by John F. Thie, D.C. with Mary Marks. De Vorss and Co., Marina del Rey, Calif., 1973. Manual to muscle testing with holistic health remedies for weaknesses.

For information on teachers trained in the Iyengar method, write Institute for Yoga Teacher Education, 1952 Lombard, San Francisco, Calif. 94123. (415) 346-2982.

Index

Poses
(By Areas of Body)

Poses
(Alphabetically)